Cure Your Allergies

Martin F. Healy Lic.Ac. (UK) MBAcC.

Cure Your Allergies

And Live Your Life

Index Compiled by Charmian Parkin

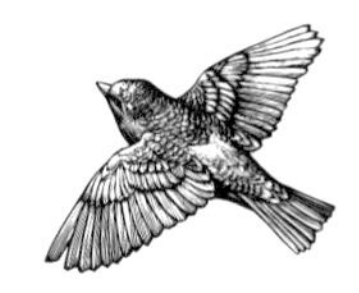

SAFFRON WALDEN
THE C.W. DANIEL COMPANY LIMITED

First published in Great Britain in 2001
by The C.W. Daniel Company Limited
1 Church Path, Saffron Walden,
Essex CB10 1JP, United Kingdom

ISBN 0 85207 347 X

Designed by Jane Norman
Produced in association with Book Production Consultants plc,
25–27 High Street, Chesterton, Cambridge CB4 1ND
Typeset by Cambridge Photosetting Services
Printed and bound by Saxon Group, Norwich

About The Author

Martin Healy studied for three years at the College of Traditional Acupuncture, England, graduating in 1983. He trained under Professor J.R. Worsley, who pioneered the use of Five Element acupuncture. Healy is a member of the British Acupuncture Council.

After graduation Martin Healy studied with Dr. Anthony Hodson, a pioneer researcher into allergy medicine in England. Since then he has worked almost exclusively with allergy patients, using a variety of tests before opting for a particular IgG blood antibody test. Five Element acupuncture provides the other element of his unique approach.

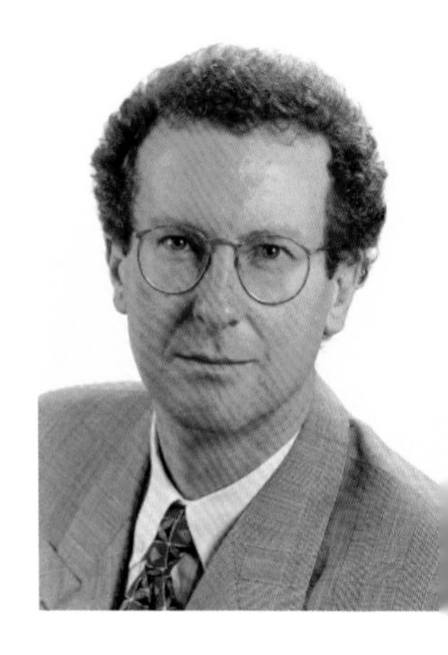

Contents

Acknowledgements

A special thank you to my teacher, Professor J.R. Worsley, who did so much to impress upon me how the root of most Western illnesses lies buried within our troubled emotions. A teacher who presented his teachings with such absolute elegance.

To Dr. Anthony Hodson a special thank you for he also had been a gracious and willing teacher. Hodson who spent his professional life "in search of a suspected something missing in the understanding of modern medicine and its dependence on drug therapy", finally came to recognise that diet was that missing something.

To his son Philip who introduced me to Dr. Hodson, thank you. Philip and I studied at acupuncture college together, and later with his father. We learned so much over those early years and got the chance to put it all into practice at his Cambridge clinic in the mid 1980s. A special friend.

To Edward Bach (1886–1936) of the Bach flower remedies fame – a man whose writings I stumbled across many years ago, and someone I have come to deeply admire. A man whose insights into the divine nature of human life and whose clarity as to the real reason for man's existence on this earth, offers Western medicine something it has never had – a philosophy.

To my very good friend and fellow practitioner Simon Charles whose indomitable spirit remains an inspiration and whose friendship has remained as constant as the northern star.

To special friends such as Maureen Gilbert, Helen Litton and Michael

Dunne, whose editing skills helped bring shape to this book. To Philip Quested, the artist who did the illustrations for this book, thank you.

To my secretary, Kate Kirwan, a special thank you, for in addition to managing the day to day running of the practice, she unselfishly encouraged and supported me during those busy two years I spent writing this book.

To all my many patients for their support over the past seventeen years, a particular thank you. Especially so to those who kindly agreed to let me use their case histories and photographs so that others may be helped just as they have been.

Both author and publisher are grateful to the Bournemouth News and Picture Agency for loan and permission to use their photograph of Patrick Webster, the record sneezer who sneezed 700 times a day for 35 years and to Craig Stennant, Otley, West Yorkshire, for the photograph of Christine Alden.

Finally, my grateful thanks to Don Harper, a great guy who went out of his way to help me when I arrived at his office with nothing more than a bundle of papers and ideas.

Introduction

In our increasingly busy world, more and more people – men, women, teenagers and even babies – are suffering from food allergies. We are all familiar with the health warnings associated with the excessive consumption of foods such as salt, fat, sugar etc. However, it is a revelation to many people that the most common allergenic foods – foods which provoke allergic reactions – are those very items which we have been advised are healthiest for us: high-fibre breakfast cereals, wholemeal bread, calcium-rich dairy products, vitamin-rich citrus fruit, and many more. For certain people, allergies to these everyday foods can be the cause of many common medical conditions, such as asthma, eczema, arthritis, migraine, sinusitis and irritable bowel syndrome.

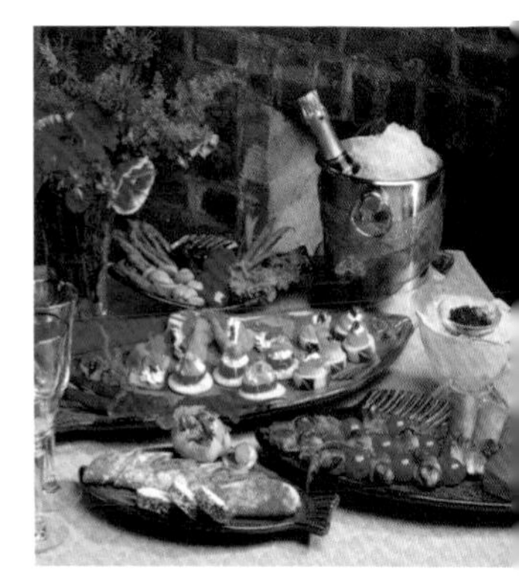

This book has been written to inform you of a new understanding of allergies based on the fact that evidence is now emerging that the majority of food allergy reactions are delayed, sometimes taking several days to manifest.

This new evidence is in stark contrast to what was believed hitherto. It also means that many of the tests that were developed prior to this understanding are now obsolete.

This book details my approach to treating allergies and how it has helped many of my patients over nearly twenty years. It pays particular attention to:

- How and why people become allergic;
- The differences between the available allergy tests;
- How to increase resistance to allergies.

This book also deals with the limitations of the applications of allergy testing. Many conditions are entirely unrelated to allergies and thus cannot be resolved by allergy testing. The case histories in this book present symptoms and conditions which, in my experience, have in general responded well to my particular approach of allergy testing, dietary change and acupuncture. For while the basic principles of dealing with allergy-related illness are the same, to get the best results, treatment should be tailored to the individual's needs.

It is hoped that this book will encourage other practitioners to consider the possibilities of the new IgG allergy test, by means of which it is now possible to identify what are called "delayed-response" allergens. However, because the available scientific evidence concerning such allergy reactions is inconclusive, the hypotheses in this book rely largely on assessment of the presenting problems of my patients. More systematic research into these issues is urgently required.

Martin F. Healy.

CHAPTER ONE

The Potential of This System

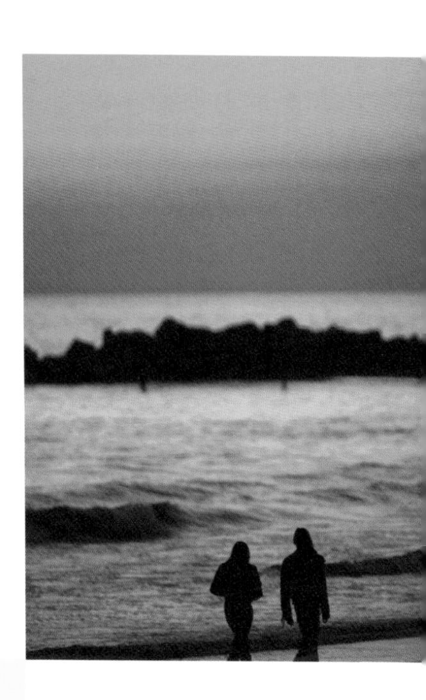

It is my belief that many of the illnesses which are at present considered to be separate medical conditions – for example, irritable bowel syndrome, asthma, eczema, psoriasis, arthritis, sinusitis and migraine – are in fact nothing more than different manifestations of the same phenomenon: food allergy. If the allergenic foods can be identified accurately, and then removed from the diet, there is very often a significant improvement in health.

Most affected people have relatively few primary allergies – two or three at most – so the process of allergy identification is rarely onerous. Improvement can usually be seen within days of starting an appropriately modified diet, and certainly in less than three weeks.

The following two extracts from recent newspaper articles give an indication of what is possible. They are particularly relevant because the people concerned allowed their identity to be known, and openly shared with readers every aspect of their condition and the outcome after treatment.

The symptoms described in these articles are the symptoms most commonly presented by allergy sufferers. If your particular complaint is similar to these, it is likely that you can expect a similar outcome.

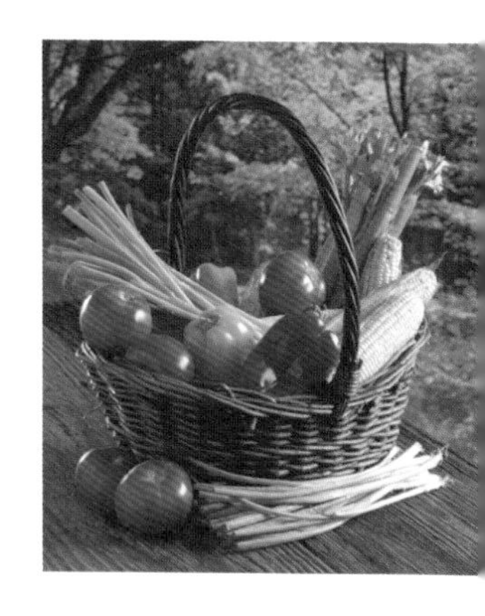

The Irish Times, Monday, *January 11, 1999*

New allergy tests may mean an end to long lists of forbidden foods – and better results. Already, one Dublin specialist is combining them with acupuncture to combat the side-effects of the pace of life. **Arminta Wallace** *was impressed.*

Why do so many people seem to suffer from allergies nowadays? Twenty years ago you weren't considered to have an allergy unless you dropped dead at the sight of a cat or keeled over after eating shellfish. Now, every self-respecting household seems to have somebody who's allergic to something; dust mite, cows' milk, dog hair, gluten, yeast, cashew nuts ... the list is apparently endless. Is allergy somehow connected to economic prosperity? Is it a product of our diet, with its emphasis on processed foods? Or is it simply something dreamed up by middle-class folk who have nothing better to think about?

According to Martin Healy, clinical director of the Fitzwilliam Acupuncture and Allergy Clinic, a specialist in allergy studies (...). "In traditional societies allergy and allergy-related illness is virtually unknown, because people work at a less rushed pace", he says. "Allergy people are busy, busy people who work at 100 miles an hour, under constant pressures, subject to constant deadlines. They often complain they can't eat this or that any more, whereas up to a few years ago they hadn't an ache or a pain and could eat stones."

Obviously, however, the patients who turn up at Martin Healy's door are not imagining their illnesses. Many have suffered for years from asthma, eczema, irritable bowel conditions, migraine, or just a general feeling of "unwellness". So, what is making them unwell? Time, perhaps to make the acquaintance of the autonomic nervous system.

"This is the system which controls digestion, "as Healy explains. (...)" The autonomic nervous system can be regarded as an intelligence which orchestrates the entire digestive process." It is also intimately bound up with the emotions – so when the system is subject to persistent heavy doses of stress, it is weakened to the point where it can no longer process certain foods. "That's what a food allergy is; it's a food which stays in the gut undigested. The majority of allergy people talk about tummy upsets, bloated feelings, indigestion – these are all triggered by undigested food poisoning the system. And the more we stress and hassle ourselves, the more we weaken the autonomic nervous system, to the point where it doesn't recognise and can't process the culprit foods, which is why allergies are becoming more prevalent." (...)

As for the physical results of all this stress and bother, Healy paints a grim picture. "When food is not digested it begins to curdle and become toxic. If an egg goes off, or milk goes sour, think of how it smells – now think of that inside your body." (...)

This reporter's trial test showed up a fairly serious allergy to dairy products and eggs, something of a shock result for someone who, having been down the irritable bowel/stomach ulcer/early-morning-queasiness road for many years, had taken to drinking vast quantities of milk and eating mountains of scrambled egg in a misguided attempt to improve the digestive situation.

One dairy-free month later the early-morning queasiness has completely vanished and there have been no unpleasant stomach "episodes" at all. No more ice cream, either; but when you feel 100 per cent better, you don't argue with that.

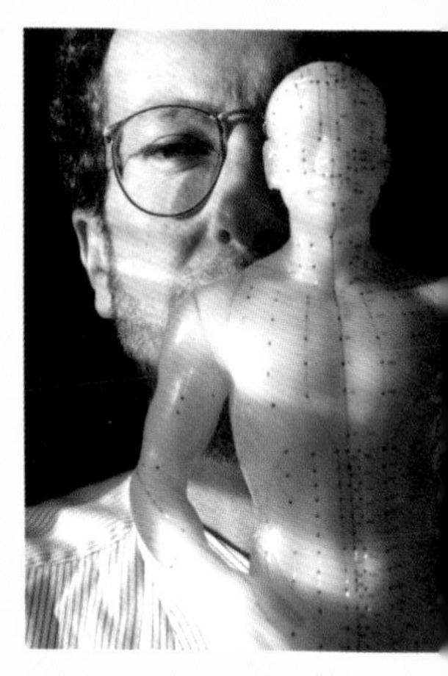

Michael Kennedy [name changed] is a 17-year-old school student from (...) Co. Kildare. He had suffered from continuous colds and flu which led to breathlessness – a major problem as he is a promising athlete. About a year ago he developed a serious bout of pneumonia, which cleared after treatment with antibiotics but left him weak and demoralised; he also continued to suffer from low-grade colds. The allergy test showed that Michael had one very serious food allergy and a minor reaction to two other foods. Within a week of avoiding these foods he felt better; his chest began to clear, his energy returned and he was able to train with an enthusiasm which had been missing for two years.

Helen O'Sullivan [name changed] is a 47-year-old married woman from Co. Cork. For twenty years she had been under constant medical care for various chronic problems including an irritable-bowel-like condition which led to headaches, asthma, skin rashes and weight gain. She also suffered from hyper attacks which would come on without warning, triggering serious bouts of high blood pressure and leave her shaking all over. Her laboratory report suggested she suffered from two serious allergies; she avoided the foods concerned, and within two weeks all her symptoms disappeared. Six months after being tested, she remains in excellent health.

(Reproduced by kind permission of The Irish Times, Monday, January 11, 1999.)

Photo courtesy of Frank Miller, The Irish Times

The Big Issues *(Eire), Issue 117, April 14, 1999*

Rosemarie Meleady* *reports on a new procedure, which is set to cause a stir in health circles – a simple allergy test which you can quickly identify if you are suffering as a result of food intolerance.*

Martin Healy, clinical director of the Fitzwilliam Acupuncture and Allergy Clinic, approached me two months ago about trying out a simple test he is using to cure people of common complaints such as irritable bowel, eczema, migraine, etc. It was strange because he called on my mother's birthday and the ideal gift for her would be to restore her health.

My mother suffers from severe sinus trouble – by severe I mean she gets up in the morning and starts to sneeze until midday; at around dinner time she would again start to sneeze and could continue sneezing through the night. When I say sneeze, I mean eye-popping forceful sneezes. Often she would sneeze for 48 hours, hardly without a break.

She tried everything from aura cleansing to Chinese remedies but nothing stopped it. Her face would be constantly swollen, her eyes streamed and the strong medication her GP had her on to suppress the sneezing, would make her sleepy. This had been going on for about twenty years and now that my mother is in her 60s there were concerns how this constant, exhausting sneezing would affect her heart. She has also suffered from indigestion problems and irritable bowel for as long as she can remember.

So when Healy invited me to send someone on a trial to his clinic I immediately thought of my mother and booked her in.

According to Healy, the main problem for allergy patients is that their immune systems are over-reacting to harmless substances, such as pollens, and innocent foods, such as dairy products. It is producing "all out attack" antibodies in response to these innocent products. These antibodies should only be used against serious bacterial or viral invasion.

It took 10 days for my mother's results to come back. The report showed a strong reaction to wheat and yeast, with cows' milk, eggs and legumes (beans and peas) giving a mild reaction. My mother has always made her own bread with wheat germ, bran and all these things which she thought would help her digestion problem when in fact, in her case, these were causing all her health problems.

Three days after ruling these out of her diet she could already see an improvement in her health – she was sleeping much better and wasn't getting her daily bout of indigestion. One week later there were dramatic improvements, with bonuses! Her indigestion had completely gone, she was no longer feeling bloated, she was sleeping much more soundly and the nightmares she experienced nightly since childhood had stopped.

Two weeks after starting the "diet" my mother received her first acupuncture treatment from Martin. She rang me the next morning, exclaiming that for the first time in years she slept breathing through her nose. This may not seem to be a big achievement but it meant she did not wake up with a dry mouth and throat which led to a rasping cough and it also meant that my father was not kept awake by her snoring!

A few days after her second treatment of acupuncture she stopped taking the strong suppressive medication her GP had been prescribing her for 17 years – a month has since passed and she hasn't sneezed once. I now see a different woman. Her eyes are no longer puffy, her face has a healthy glow rather than blotchy and swollen, she is of a much healthier weight.

For the first time in her life she could smell the flowers I got her for Mother's Day.

** Rosemarie Meleady is Editor of The Big Issues magazine.*
(Reproduced by kind permission of The Big Issues, April 14, 1999.)

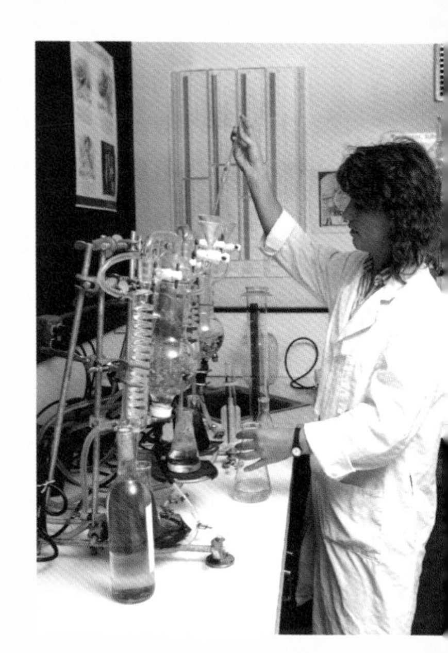

Allergy and Stress

It has been my experience that in the majority of cases, the ultimate causative factor in allergies is emotional distress resulting from excessive worry and stress.

There is a body of opinion which blames the prevalence of allergy-related illness on such things as pollution, central heating, processed food, household pets and carpets. I believe such things to be secondary or associated factors. The ultimate factor, which I believe to be at the root of the enormous increase in allergy-related conditions over the past 20 years, is **the competitiveness, the rushing and racing and all the other stresses which have become an integral part of modern Western society.**

Resulting stress leads to emotional problems which disrupt individuals' nervous systems and subsequently their immune systems to the point where they become over-sensitive to their everyday foods and environment.

The treatment approach recommended throughout this book involves a particular allergy test which has been designed to detect those foods which are causing intestinal toxicity. This dietary approach has as its primary objective the maintenance of good intestinal health.

In addition to dealing with the allergies I have incorporated Five Element Acupuncture into my overall treatment approach. This style of acupuncture is particularly helpful for medical conditions which have a strong emotional association. It strengthens the nervous system, enabling it to manage better the emotional load which is being placed upon it.

Chapter Two

The Immune System

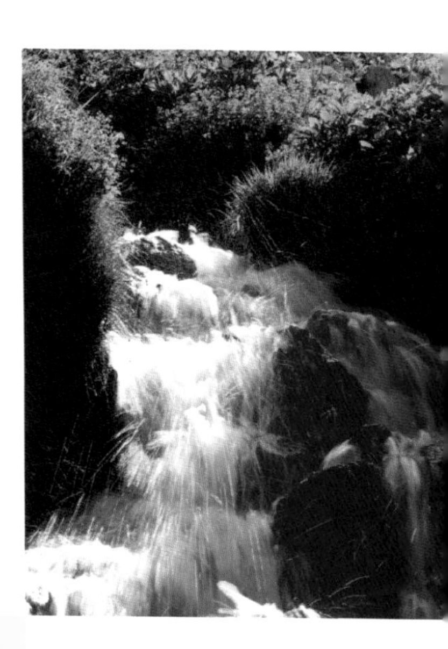

Allergies are associated with an imbalance in the immune system. The immune system is a highly complex system, but only those aspects which relate to allergies need be discussed here.

The immune system defends the body from attack by harmful bacteria or viruses. When it is working well it also protects us from developing either food or environmental allergies. It is responsible for all repair and healing that takes place within the body. We commonly hear people say that they are very prone to catching colds and that when they do they are very slow in shaking them off. What happens is that their immune systems fail to protect them from cold viruses in the air, and when the cold begins, their immune systems are also ineffective at dealing with and curing the condition.

The same principle applies to allergies. When the immune system malfunctions, we are prone to developing allergies, and, equally, it is much harder to stop such allergic reactions.

Components of the Immune System

The immune system has what we might call several departments, each there to deliver a different kind of defence response. How the body responds to any particular invader – bacteria, virus or allergy – is very complex, and many of the mechanisms involved are not fully understood. However, what we do know is that the immune system has two completely separate ways of dealing with allergy-related problems. One creates an acute inflammation which triggers diarrhoea or vomiting to flush the allergy-provoking intruder out of the body as quickly as possible. The other creates intense and often chronic inflammation around the allergen in order to incinerate it.

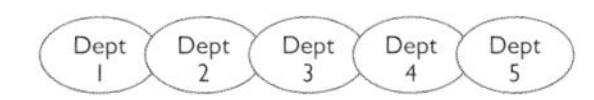

Antibodies

To communicate with these separate departments, and to activate them and trigger them into action, the immune system uses a series of antibodies. Of the five antibodies associated with the immune system, two are concerned primarily with allergies. These are IgE and IgG antibodies.

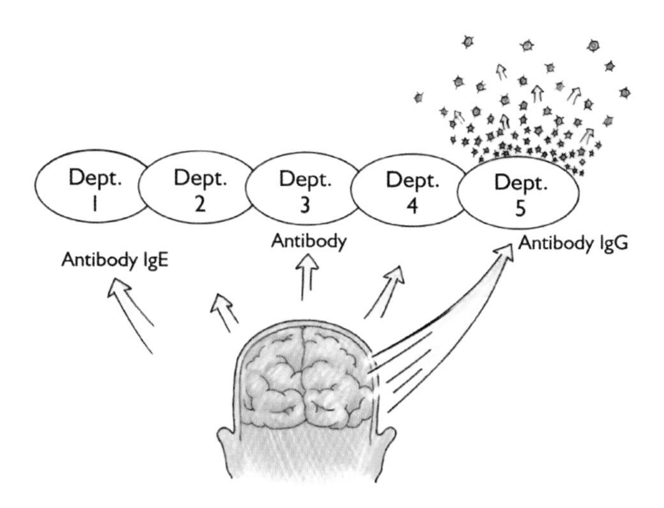

The IgE antibody: triggers an immediate inflammatory response which helps to flush allergens out of the body as quickly as possible.

The IgG antibody: takes a certain time to gather together all the forces of the immune system and then delivers a powerful inflammatory response to toxins which have entered the bloodstream. Consequently, this inflammatory response is delayed.

These delayed-response allergies are the subject of this book.

Two Main Types of Allergy Reaction

The following case histories illustrate the differences between reactions to allergens triggered by the IgE and by the IgG antibodies.

IgE Classic Allergy Reaction

Mary has had allergy tendencies all her life. As a baby she suffered from colic and had eczema on her face and hands. There was a strong family history of allergies. On her father's side, asthma was a common complaint, and on her mother's side, hayfever predominated.

As Mary grew older, she developed a mild form of asthma which was controlled by the daily use of inhalers. While she was studying for her final examinations at university, she became violently sick with vomiting and diarrhoea; her mouth and tongue swelled and she had to be rushed to hospital. This happened immediately after eating a meal in a restaurant.

The hospital did an allergy test and diagnosed that she was highly allergic to shellfish. Mary realised that she had had prawns as a starter with her lunch and that her tongue had started swelling even before she had finished the main course.

She was advised that this type of allergy reaction remains for life and that if ever she ate shellfish again, it was possible that the next reaction could be even more severe and possibly smother her. She was also advised to carry a special adrenaline pen so that she could inject herself immediately if ever she found her tongue swelling as a result of inadvertently eating shellfish. By scrupulously avoiding shellfish she has remained well ever since.

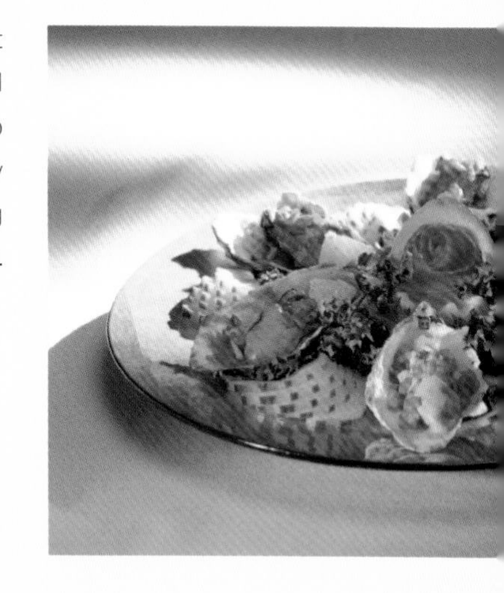

IgG Delayed-response Allergy Reaction

Pat enjoyed very good health for much of his life. Now in his mid-forties, he was appointed manager of a local bank two years ago. For the past year his health has been deteriorating. He has been suffering with irritable bowel syndrome, manifesting as bloating and cramping within the intestines. He is also very tired for much of the time: no matter how much he sleeps, he is never really refreshed for long. His sinus passages are becoming blocked, causing headaches and migraine-type pains across his temples and forehead.

His doctor has tried every investigation possible but nothing specific has shown up. A specialist recommended a high fibre diet for the irritable bowel problem but this only made matters worse. He has a steroid spray for his sinusitis, but it gives only temporary relief and he is also worried about possible long-term effects. He has had three courses of antibiotics already this year for the sinusitis, and the relief they give is shorter with each course. In summer his eyes burn and itch and he fears he is now beginning to suffer with hayfever.

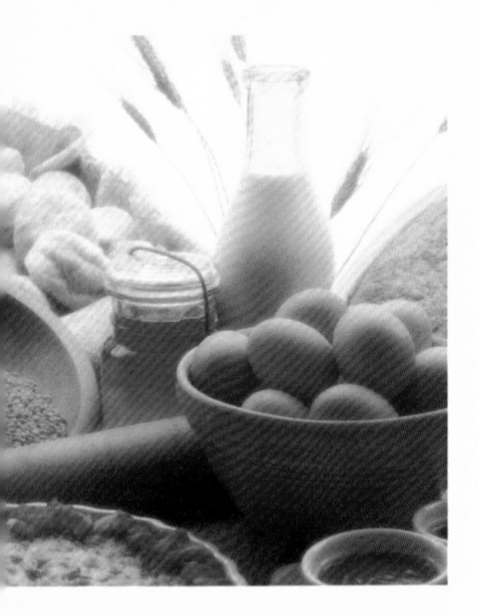

Pat decided to have his blood tested for delayed-response IgG allergies. The results indicated a strong reaction to three foods: dairy products, beef and eggs. At the end of the first week of avoiding these foods there was a remarkable improvement. The irritable bowel problem had completely cleared up and returned to normal functioning. By the end of the second week, not only had the sinusitis cleared up but the migraine was almost gone. His energy was back and his zest for life and work had also returned.

Important Differences Between the Two Reactions

There are clear differences between the two allergic reactions. Mary's allergy, which causes an immediate reaction, is well-documented in medical texts and is familiar to the majority of people.

By contrast, the main feature of Pat's allergy reactions, which made it difficult for his own GP to diagnose, was the fact that he was not showing symptoms immediately after eating the offending foods. The symptoms were building over a period of time as the allergic foods slowly poisoned his system, causing intense inflammation at various sites. This is "delayed response food allergy".

This type of allergy reaction is rarely discussed in medical texts and is unfamiliar to the majority of people. However, a body of evidence is now emerging which suggests that the majority of foods which trigger allergy reactions involve this slow poisoning process (1).

As yet there is no universally accepted term for the different types of reactions. Usually the term "allergy" is used for fast reactions, while slow reactions are termed "sensitivity" or "intolerance". Throughout this book a combination of terms is used but in all cases, unless otherwise stated, it is slow- or delayed-response allergies (sensitivities) that are being discussed.

The IgE Antibody

The most important characteristic of the IgE antibody is that it stores a memory of each invader. It has intelligence and the potential to learn. This means that the antibody can carry out a more thorough attack on the allergen each time it re-encounters it. The great danger with this lies in reactions which produce a swelling of the tongue, lips or the throat. It is very likely that as the antibody learns to produce a better attack response, the next encounter with the trigger may result in a more severe reaction.

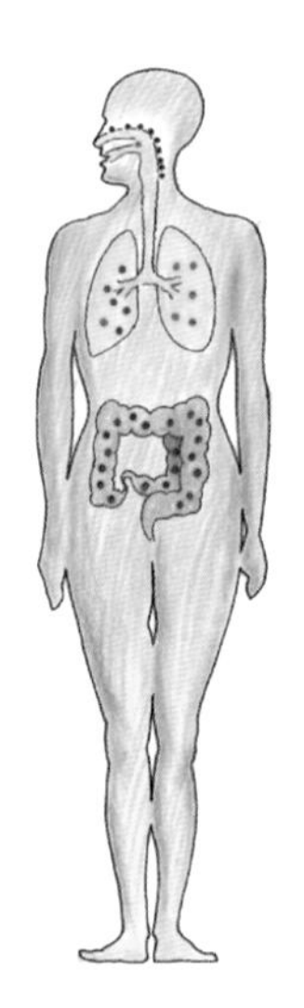

Diagram 1

How the IgE Antibody Works

Mast cells are special sacs which contain protective chemicals. They are embedded in tissues located around the nose and in the lungs, skin and intestines (see Diagram 1). At these sites they are well positioned to guard the body's vulnerable entrance points from invaders.

The IgE antibody is attached to the surface of these mast cells somewhat like an antenna (see Diagram 2).

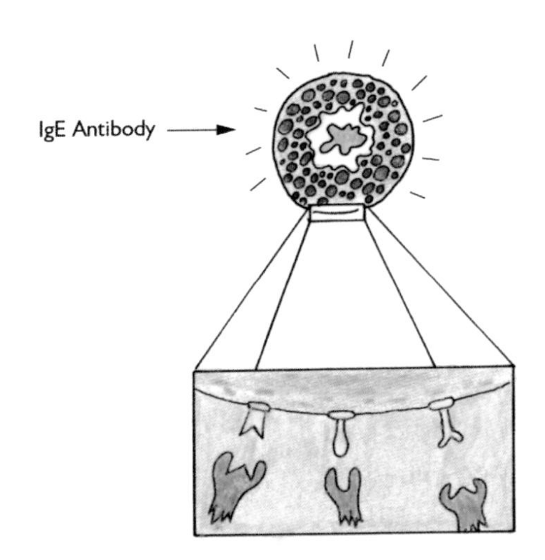

Diagram 2 Microscopic view of antibody attached to surface of mast cell

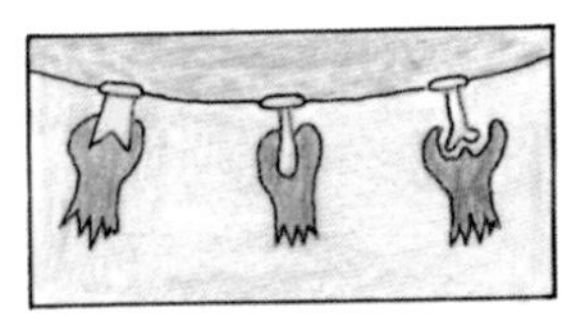

Diagram 3a

Once an allergic trigger touches the antibody (see Diagram 3a), it signals to the mast cell the command to release its chemical contents (see Diagram 3b), causing chaos in the surrounding tissues. One of the main chemicals released is histamine, hence the use of drugs named antihistamines to counteract its effects. Histamine is an enzyme that triggers all the classic symptoms of allergy, including:

- coughing and sneezing;
- streaming eyes and nose;

- vomiting;
- diarrhoea;
- swelling of the tissues.

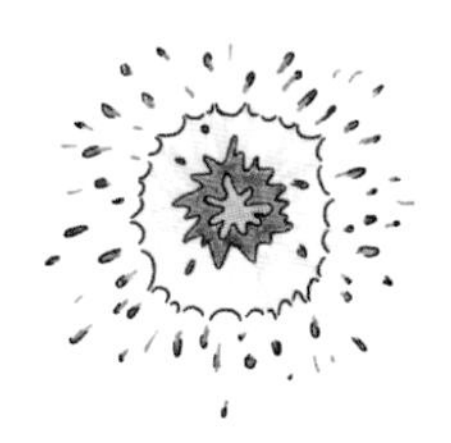

Diagram 3b

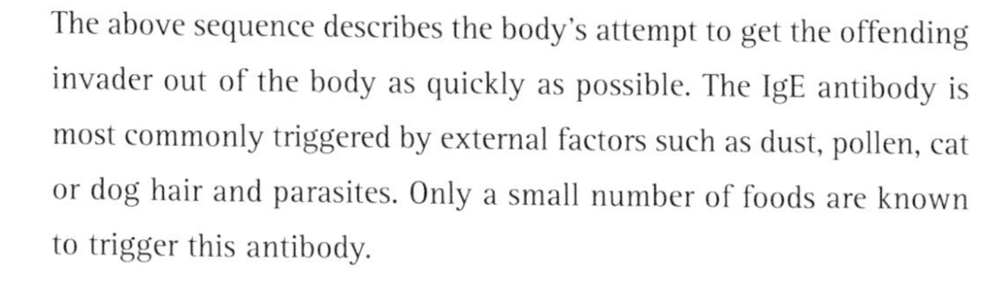

The above sequence describes the body's attempt to get the offending invader out of the body as quickly as possible. The IgE antibody is most commonly triggered by external factors such as dust, pollen, cat or dog hair and parasites. Only a small number of foods are known to trigger this antibody.

Because of this immediate reaction, the majority of people suffering from IgE antibody allergies are able to recognise their own trigger agents and seldom need to resort to specific allergy tests.

The IgG Antibody

The IgG antibody is primarily concerned with toxins, many of which are manufactured within the intestines and make their way into the bloodstream. One way in which the IgG antibody works is to search out such toxins and attach itself to their surface (2). Doing this, it attracts the most powerful inflammatory cells of the immune system, directing them to attack whatever it is attached to. Heat and intense inflammation are by-products of the attack.

The IgG antibody has the following predominant characteristics:

- It activates a major defence response.
- It attempts to neutralise the invader by creating intense inflammation in the area concerned.
- The reactions which result from the IgG antibody take two to three days to manifest, making it almost impossible for individuals to trace which particular foods are making them ill.

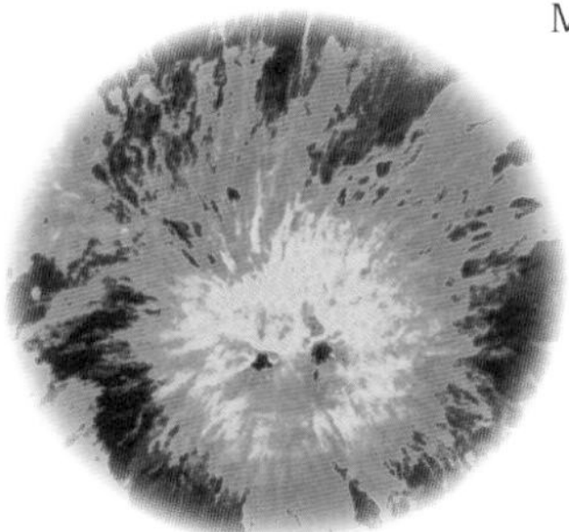

Many of our most common chronic conditions are in principle to be suspected of being associated with this antibody. Conditions where such symptoms of inflammation as heat, redness, pain and swelling are the outstanding features, and which cannot be directly associated with an injury or obvious infection, should be investigated with this in mind.

Detecting the Type of Allergy

Much of the confusion relating to allergies stems from the lack of understanding of the delayed reaction outlined above.

Most allergy tests are designed to detect IgE antibody allergy reactions. The IgE antibody was discovered in the 1960s and is relatively well researched and understood. However, because the majority of food allergens do not activate the IgE antibody process, the allergy tests come back negative. As a result, the tendency has been to deny the existence of most food allergies.

It is only in the past few years that research has shown how the IgG antibody marker controls the delayed allergy reaction (3). Such research promises to revolutionize the practice of allergy medicine.

Chapter Three

How Food Allergies Begin

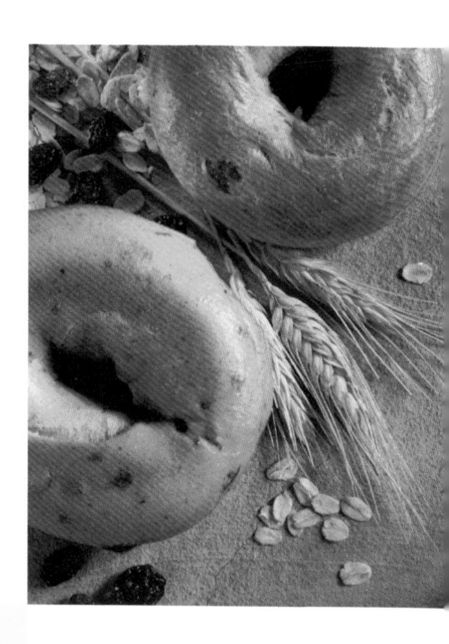

The body cannot use any food unless it has first broken it down into its simplest component parts. To do this, foods trigger a series of digestive glands into producing a measured amount of digestive enzyme. For example:

- **Fats** trigger the gallbladder to secrete bile in order to dissolve and break down the fat as it passes through the digestive system.
- **Sugars** trigger the insulin glands to produce insulin in order to help with the breakdown and the absorption of sugar as it passes through the system.

The working of the digestive glands is controlled by the autonomic nervous system (see Diagram 4). According to Professor J.A. Brostoff, reader of Clinical Immunology at University College London Medical School, "thanks to the action of the autonomic nervous system, any disorder of the digestive system can be exacerbated by the emotions" (4). Worry and stress can overload these autonomic nerves, causing the digestive system to malfunction and lose the ability to co-ordinate the proper digestion of food. This results in undigested foods arriving in the intestines. These undigested foods ultimately become allergic foods.

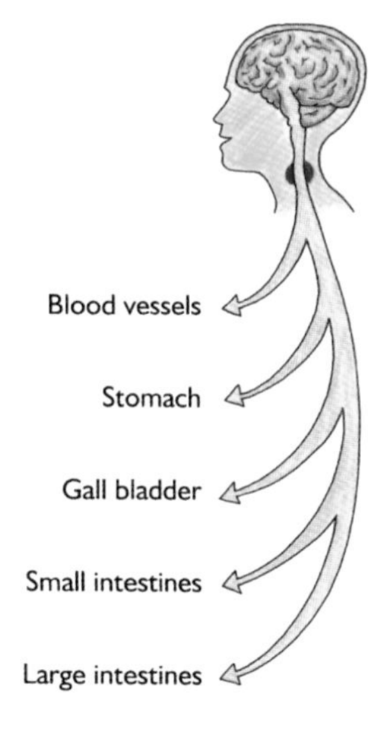

Diagram 4

Our digestive system may be thought of as a hollow tube which runs the entire length of the body. As partially digested food passes down the intestinal tract, nutrients are absorbed, mostly from the small intestine. The ability of the intestinal tract to absorb nutrients while at the same time blocking entry to toxins is dependent upon the healthy functioning of its very sensitive lining. If excessively high levels of particular toxins are present, such as certain drugs, alcohol or undigested foods, the sensitive intestinal lining can be damaged. This can result in the absorption of toxins and undigested food particles into the person's system.

How Food Allergies Develop

Over time, the continuous consumption of allergic food leads to a build-up of toxins within the intestines. Should these toxins eventually make their way into the bloodstream, they are then carried by the blood throughout the body (5). Once in circulation, they can affect other organs and body systems (6).

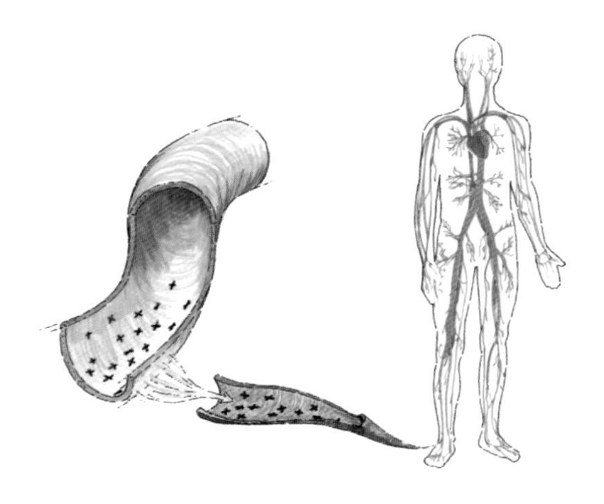

The immune system responds to this toxic invasion of the blood by activating the IgG antibodies, and this marks the beginning of the person's inflammatory-allergic response.

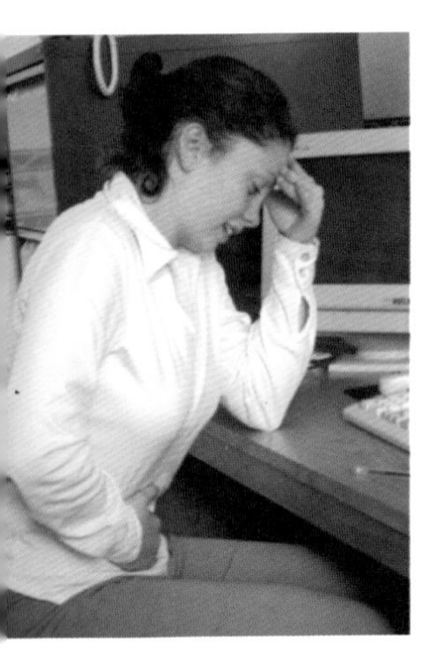

Symptoms of Food Allergy

Intestinal upset is common to most food allergy sufferers, whose symptoms may include:

- Flatulence;
- Bloating;
- Indigestion;
- "Nervous stomach";
- Diarrhoea or constipation.

Only recently has it been acknowledged scientifically that toxins within the intestinal tract can adversely affect health. Many of the "nature cure treatments" of our grandparents' time proposed that body toxicity lay at the root of many illnesses. Advocates of these were for the most part unable to explain the exact mechanism which led to toxicity but were clear about directing treatment towards clearing these toxins from the body. They used a combination of fasting and herbs to purge the bowel and cleanse the blood. We can now see the wisdom in many of these old natural cures; but with a better understanding of bowel toxicity and its role in allergies, we can now provide more accurately targeted treatments.

How Toxins Trigger Disease

Alan Ebringer, while professor of Immunology at King's College, University of London, explained inflammatory reaction in relation to rheumatoid arthritis. His research indicated that in certain cases of this disease, toxins which originate in the bowel are able to trick the immune system into attacking its own joints. Dr. Ebringer found that in certain people the cell structure of these toxins is very similar to the cell structure of the protective covering of their joints. In such people, if these toxins escape out of the bowel into the bloodstream, the immune system responds by sending out IgG antibodies to attack them. However, the antibodies mistake the protective covering on the joints for the toxins and begin to attack the joints, often quite aggressively.

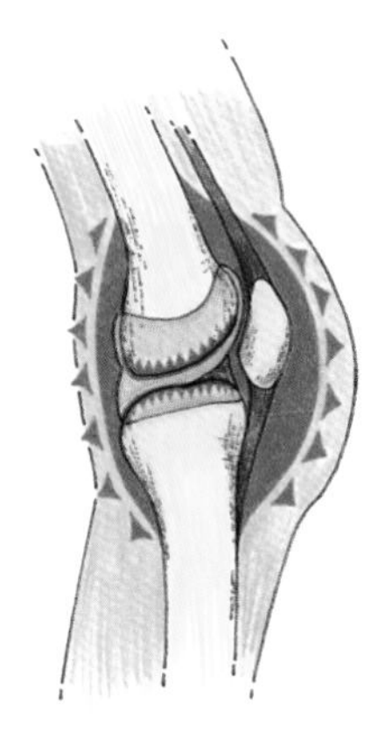

This mechanism may well be involved in other inflammatory and autoimmune diseases, especially those which respond to the allergy approach. By finding the allergy foods and eliminating them from the diet, bowel toxins can be dealt with before they can enter the bloodstream. As a result, the immune system stops its attack upon the affected body part.

Other inflammatory conditions which commonly respond well to the allergy approach include irritable bowel syndrome, asthma, arthritis, migraine, sinusitis and many skin conditions.

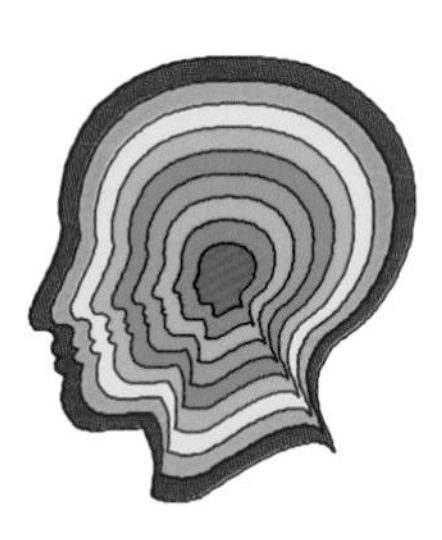

"Antibody Mistakes"

We know that the autonomic nerves transmit the effects of emotional change, including stress and worry, throughout the body (7). We also know that there are autonomic nerve connections to the lymphatic centres, where these antibodies are manufactured and "programmed" (8).

Given this, it seems very likely that these autonomic nerves allow the effects of stress somehow to be encoded into antibodies, causing them to malfunction. This causes the IgE antibody to over-react to pollen, house-dust, shellfish and the like, and the IgG antibody to attack body tissue which is similar in cell structure to that of a toxin.

The reason why I believe stress is at the root of these allergy reactions is because in so many cases, acupuncture treatment directed towards easing the emotional turmoil of the patient, considerably reduces these allergy-inflammatory reactions.

Weekly News, UK *Edition No. 7, 1999*

Single drop of blood transformed her life

Drinking milk every day brought Heidi Sawyer 20 years of misery. The "pinta" she thought was doing her good was actually triggering the psoriasis, eczema and lethargy which was ruining her life.

But now, the 26-year-old has seen her health transformed by a single drop of blood.

"I've had trouble with eczema and psoriasis ever since I was a kid," explained Heidi. "It mainly affected my hands and was really bad – red, ugly-looking and painful. I tried every cream under the sun and was always at the doctors."

"In addition, I felt tired and lethargic all the time. I never seemed to have any energy and at work, I'd be nodding off in the afternoon".

"And because I had no energy to exercise, my weight shot up till I reached 12 stones".

The breakthrough came when Heidi's dad, who, convinced her diet was responsible for her troubles, pressured her to take the test.

"I couldn't believe the report when it came back showing I had severe intolerance to dairy products," said Heidi, a promotions agency account manager.

"It also showed I was intolerant to tomatoes, black pepper and kidney beans, which were in the sauces I regularly ate."

Heidi set about making the diet changes needed. She cut out the suspect substances and concentrated on plain meat, fish, vegetables and fruit. She reckons that in just two weeks she felt major benefits and within a month her sore and unsightly skin problems had cleared.

"It really was amazing," added Heidi. "I'd had years of being self-conscious and embarrassed and suddenly it has gone. My weight started coming down and down till I'd lost two and a half stones."

"Now I just feel so much better, it's been a wonderful change in my life."

(Reproduced by kind permission of Weekly News, UK. Edition No. 7, 1999.)

CHAPTER FOUR

The Causes of Bowel Toxicity

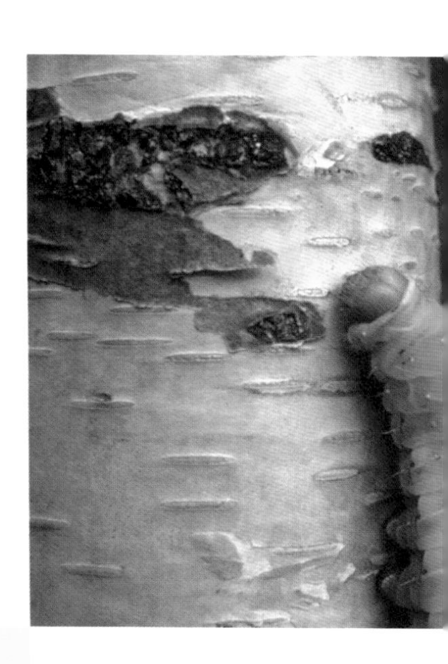

The adult digestive tract is approximately 30 feet long and, in the average person, contains up to two-and-a-half pounds of living bacteria, the majority within the large and small intestines. These bacteria can be thought of as either friendly and health-enhancing or unfriendly and toxin-producing. In good health there is a balance between the friendly and the unfriendly bacteria. If the unfriendly bacteria overwhelm and outnumber the friendly, the result is active toxins in the body (9).

Unfriendly bacteria can overwhelm friendly bacteria when:

- certain toxins and medication damage the friendly bacteria;
- the immune system becomes weakened.

One of the greatest defences against toxin-producing bacteria is to have thriving populations of friendly bacteria to oppose them. However, poisons such as insecticides, fungicides and certain medications, can damage the friendly bacteria. An overwhelming bacterial or viral attack can kill them. Long-term digestive problems and incompletely digested foods, can also weaken them. It appears that the unfriendly bacteria are far less vulnerable to these factors.

Listed below are what I consider to be the main causes of damage to these very important friendly bacteria:

Antibiotics

The appropriate use of antibiotics rarely causes problems. However, the overuse of broad-spectrum antibiotics (for example, tetracycline, minocin, ampicillin, amoxycillin) can be problematic. The damage they cause to friendly bacteria within the bowel is particularly noticeable when they are prescribed on a long-term basis, for example when tetracycline or minocin, both broad-spectrum antibiotics, are used in the treatment of acne. A passage from a current pharmacology textbook (10) describes the damage that can be done:

> *"The side effects of tetracycline are occasionally nausea, vomiting, diarrhoea, acute itching of the anus etc. Due to not being completely absorbed, part of the tetracycline reaches the bowel and destroys many of the bacteria normally present there. Certain other organisms of the yeast type, however, are not sensitive to the drug. They are therefore able to multiply profusely, resulting in a superimposed yeast infection. The yeast excretes irritant toxins which irritate the bowel and cause much intestinal upset."*

The proliferation of these yeasts within the intestines and the resultant toxins they produce then render the person concerned susceptible to developing allergic reactions.

The great worry with antibiotics is that people are becoming resistant to them. As a result, the pharmaceutical industry is forced to develop much stronger antibiotics. This is not a desirable situation for our future health (11).

Steroid Medication

Intestinal bacteria can also be disturbed by steroid drugs. The major side-effect associated with steroids is that they suppress the immune system (12). The American Food and Drug Administration requires the manufacturers of all steroids to print the following warning on the packaging of steroid drugs: "Children who are on immune-suppressant drugs are more susceptible to infection than healthy children. Chicken pox and measles, for example, can have a more serious or even fatal course in children on immune-suppressive drugs" (13). The degree of suppression depends on the strength of the prescription and the length of time it is taken.

When steroids were first introduced, they were regarded as "miracle drugs". Thousands of people who were chronically ill received a new lease of life. Associated side-effects were not recognised and they were very often prescribed in high dosages. Within a short period of time, however, a litany of side-effects began to appear, and those who thought themselves cured as a result of these steroids found that they had replaced one set of disease symptoms for another. The side-effects were often as debilitating as the disease they were intended to treat (14).

In more recent years high dosage steroids have been prescribed only for very short periods of time, usually just long enough to get the condition under control. Long-term steroids are given in very low dosages. This precaution minimises but does not completely remove the associated negative effects (15).

The Contraceptive Pill

The contraceptive pill is also a steroid drug, involving some of the complications associated with other steroids. For those who have allergic tendencies, I have observed that its use can over time exacerbate allergy reactions. Practitioners are now beginning to amass an important body of evidence on this issue (16).

Hormone Replacement Therapy (HRT)

HRT, another steroid drug, can also be a major factor in bowel bacterial disturbance. It has been my experience that for some allergy-sensitive women HRT can be the worst offender of all. As with the contraceptive pill, the symptoms take a long time to develop and, because of this, the association is often missed.

The Effect of Diet on Intestinal Bacteria

Many studies suggest a strong association of the balance between friendly and unfriendly bacteria within the intestinal tract and diet (17). The view is put forward that particular diets lead to an accumulation of excessive numbers of clostridium and other unfriendly bacteria in the intestines. The particular foods which appear to promote this intestinal toxicity are the very foods that repeatedly show positive on the allergy test.

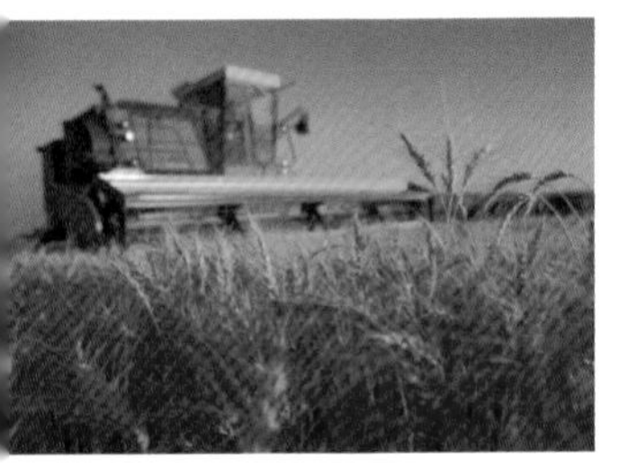

Dr. Denis Burkitt in his book *Don't Forget Fibre In Your Diet* (18), a respected reference on matters relating to diet and intestinal health, points out that many of the most common diseases of the Western world exhibit the same underlying features, including low stool bulk and a disturbance of the ratio of friendly to unfriendly bacteria within the intestinal tract.

Intestinal Bacteria and the Immune System

Antibiotics, steroid drugs, including the Contraceptive Pill and HRT, and diet all appear to be strong contributory factors in creating an imbalance between friendly and unfriendly bacteria in the human body. But we need also to recognize the part played in this by the immune system. We can say that the immune system has overall control over this balance of intestinal bacteria. It is because of their very robust and healthy immune systems that certain people can use antibiotics and steroids, and even eat badly, but still maintain a positive bacterial balance.

Immune System	
Overactive	Produces allergy reactions
Balanced	Produces the correct reaction
Underactive	Produces a weak defence response to viruses and bacteria which attack the body

We know that deficiencies in essential nutrients (vitamin C, zinc, etc.) can lead to immune system malfunction. We know that certain toxins will attack the immune system. Last but certainly not least is **the connection between the immune system and the mind.**

It is this that I believe to be the primary cause of immune system malfunction. The hypothesized connection relates to a branch of immunology known as psychoneuroimmunology. In *Say Yes To Life* (19), Dr. Clive Wood, a physiologist at the University of Oxford, explores the mind-body and mind-immune system connection, presenting a map of the connection between the nervous system and the immune system and explaining how we might imagine they communicate with each other. His view is that the way we think and feel produces specific chemical changes in the nervous system, which in turn communicates a response to the immune system. Through these connections, stress and worry will affect the immune system and cause it to malfunction.

Physicians of traditional Chinese medicine, who include an assessment of their patients' emotional disposition as an integral part of their diagnostic skills, have for thousands of years emphasised the deleterious affect of negative emotions such as worry and stress on the body's healing powers. Now medical scientists such as Dr. Wood are able to demonstrate how many of these long-held beliefs of association might be connected.

Significantly, acupuncture has been found to be capable of rebalancing the nervous system, and consequently the emotions, and, through this, of achieving an enormously positive effect upon the immune system. By combining acupuncture with the allergy test which pinpoints those toxin-forming foods, a very great deal can be achieved.

Chapter Five

Candida Albicans

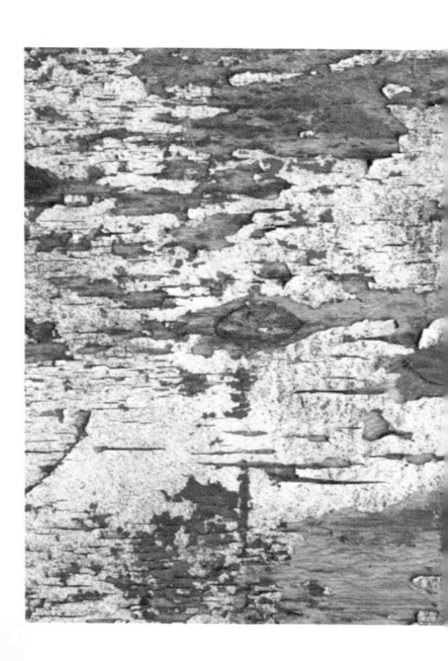

There are over four hundred different species of organism within the intestines, of which candida albicans is one. When it is kept in check by a strong immune system and by flourishing populations of healthy bacteria, candida does not pose a threat to health. A trend has emerged of associating every symptom of intestinal upset and allergy with candida. This is potentially misleading and essentially untrue.

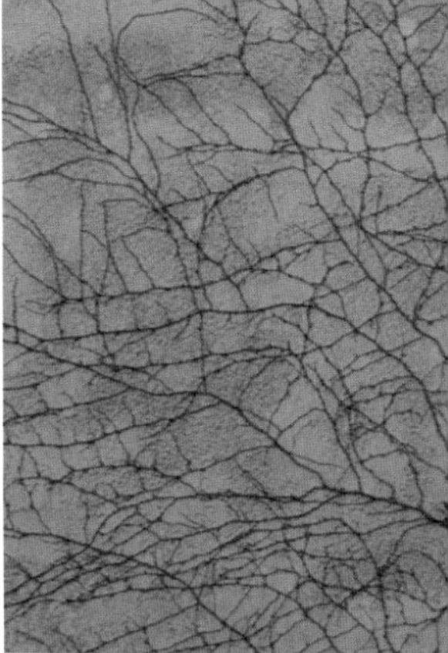

However, in some people whose immune systems are severely weakened the candida organism can dramatically increase in number within the intestinal tract. As it grows in strength, it develops characteristics which can pose a serious threat to the health of the individual:

- Toxins produced by the candida organism appear to be the most poisonous of all intestinal bacteria.
- Candida grows roots which burrow into the intestinal wall (20), increasing the latter's permeability. The existing toxins within the bowel and the additional toxins that the candida produces are then able to pass much more readily into the bloodstream, producing a poisonous state in the body.

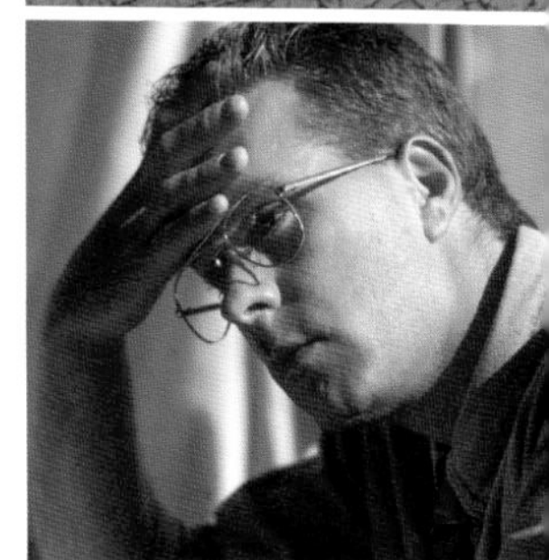

Causes of Candida Overgrowth

An increased presence of candida albicans shows that the immune system is severely compromised and weakened. As with all bowel bacterial disturbance, candida albicans overgrowth can be triggered by food allergies, antibiotics, steroids and anything else that weakens the immune system.

However, the outstanding feature which I have observed as common to people with a candida problem is extremely high levels of stress, anxiety and worry (21).

Diagnosis

The laboratory test for overgrowth of candida albicans involves a search for specific antibodies. The interpretation of this can be difficult, as candida organisms are always present, even in the healthiest bowel. During any given day, there is a constant waxing and waning of the candida organism within the bowel, and this is entirely normal. As a consequence, the detection of antibodies specific to candida albicans does not tell us very much. It simply indicates that candida albicans is present; but we already know that.

Because of this, it is important to look for features characteristically associated with this condition, notably:

- Becoming increasingly sensitive to chemicals;
- Worsening of symptoms in damp weather.

Allergic Reactions to Chemicals

Allergic reactions to chemicals are often a distinctive feature of candida overgrowth. Affected people are very sensitive to a cross-section of chemicals in their environment. It is very difficult to diagnose chemical allergies using tests available to us at present. However, because such reactions are of an immediate nature, the person concerned is often able to detect his or her own chemical allergies. Obvious examples are walking into a newly painted room and immediately feeling unwell, or applying a particular perfume or aftershave and immediately becoming asthmatic.

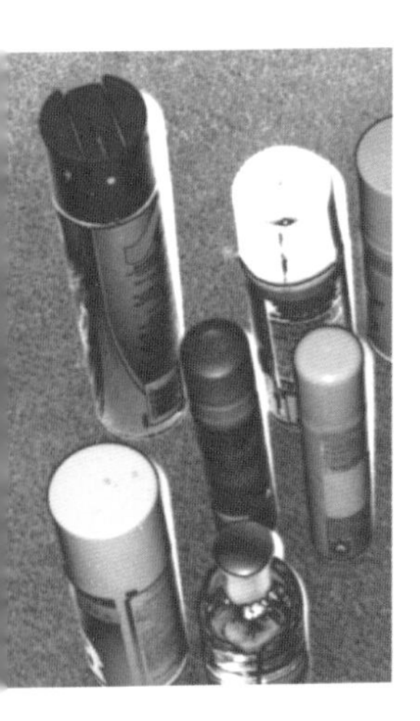

Because of the prevalence of such chemicals it has become almost impossible to avoid them completely. No list could be complete because of the vast number of chemicals used. Awareness of the major sources, however, will at least assist people in their efforts to detect their most likely trigger and to reduce their overall exposure to such chemicals.

Aerosol sprays and highly-perfumed cosmetics are obvious places to start on a campaign of reducing overall chemical exposure. Deodorants, antiperspirants, body creams, soaps and shampoos, should be replaced wherever possible with natural or fragrance-free, hypoallergenic products. Within the home, floor and furniture polishes, carpet shampoos, disinfectants and detergents, all include chemicals which can trigger allergic reactions.

Candida and Damp Weather

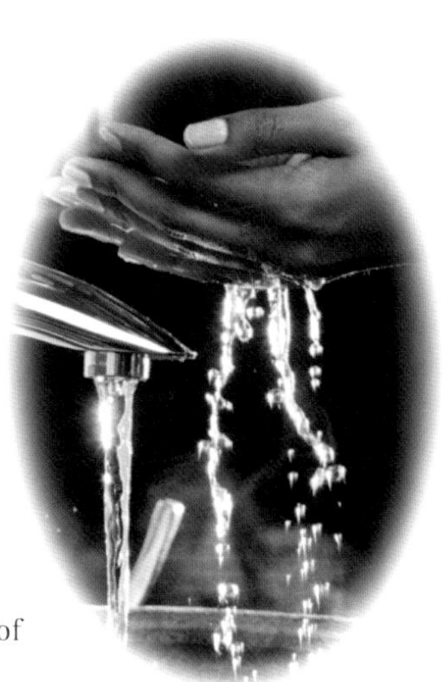

Candida albicans is a yeast, and all yeasts thrive in a damp environment. The damper the environment, the more they thrive and the more toxins they produce as a result.

The connection between this characteristic sign of candida and the fact that affected people feel noticeably better in dry climates is a pattern which I began to notice many years ago. Although there appear to be no scientific trials establishing the validity of these observations, the emerging pattern seems to score in excess of mere coincidence.

A particularly clear example involved a patient of mine who worked in financial services in London and had a very mild form of asthma. He was also sensitive to cigarette smoke and paint fumes. Interestingly he always suffered a dramatic and instant worsening of his symptoms on returning to his native city of Cork at Christmas time. He himself observed the association and recognized that the worst attacks would always coincide with particularly wet and damp weather. As soon as he began to walk down the steps from the plane at Cork airport, his asthma worsened, without fail, every year. And, within twenty-four hours of returning to London, which is colder but much drier than Cork in winter time, his symptoms would always dramatically improve.

This man was also aware of the stress aspect of his condition. He acknowledged that working in financial services was for him particularly stressful, and recognized that the symptoms were more affected by cigarette smoke and other chemicals, and also by damp weather, when his stress levels were highest.

Candida and Arthritis

To a greater or lesser degree dampness affects all allergy-related conditions. As noted above, people who suffer with allergy-related illnesses often experience a noticeable improvement in their general health when they move to a drier climate.

A condition with an obvious dampness association is arthritis. Many people with arthritis feel a definite worsening of their symptoms when the barometer falls. Some are so sensitive to dampness that they can predict when it is going to rain.

It is my belief that in such cases the approaching dampness further exacerbates an already overgrown candida situation, causing it to produce more toxins within the intestines, which then escape into the bloodstream. The inflammatory process that we associate with arthritis is then further aggravated by these toxins. Not all arthritis conditions are weather- or even allergy-related, but people who do notice a connection should consider investigating the allergy approach further.

Candida and Stress

A feature which seems to be common to candida sufferers is that they appear to be quite unaware of their high levels of stress and anxiety. Their entire focus is instead on the physical symptoms of their allergy reaction.

Opinions differ as to whether stress is the cause or the result of candida. It is my belief that it can be both. However, in the majority of cases

I believe that the affected person has a tendency towards worry or anxiety in excess of the norm and that this initiates the candida process. Then, because of the distressing symptoms associated with candida, levels of anxiety increase even further. The situation can quickly become self-perpetuating, with the anxiety acting as a catalyst to the candida and the candida in turn creating more anxiety.

Candida and Sugar

Because candida is a yeast and all yeasts are fed directly by sugar, people with a candida problem should reduce their sugar intake significantly. In addition to the sugar we get from the sugar bowl, sugar is of course present in cakes, biscuits, beer, soft drinks, ice-cream and many canned and prepared foods.

Some people exchange sugar for an artificial sweetener, such as saccharine, and this is certainly better from an allergy viewpoint. However, the most natural alternative is to use honey in moderation. A low intake of honey is normally acceptable and at least contains many essential nutrients. In many borderline cases of this kind, people have to find their own tolerance level.

Chapter Six

Babies and Children

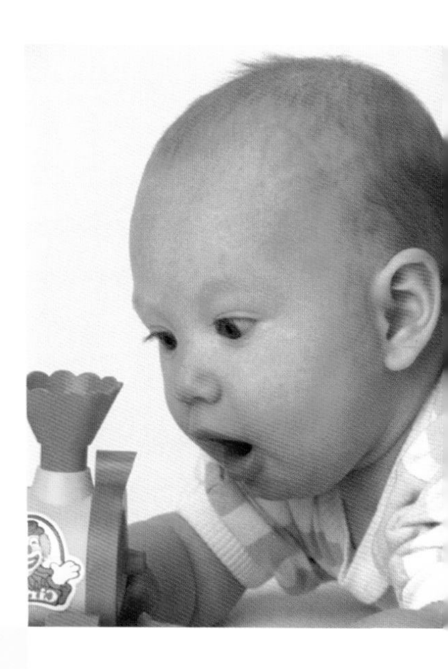

This chapter is perhaps the most important in the book because the allergy approach has the potential to assist many childhood illnesses quickly and effectively. Many people are unaware that babies and children are prone to allergies; but if the offending allergic food can be found and eliminated from the diet, their improvement is often very dramatic. Antibiotics and steroids can trigger allergies in babies and children as well as in adults.

Babies' Intestinal Flora

Unlike adults, in whom the balance between friendly and unfriendly bacteria in the gut is fairly stable, intestinal flora in infants and children can be disturbed very easily. When the unfriendly bacteria dominate, toxins appear, triggering many childhood illnesses.

For the majority of adults the bowel wall is an efficient barrier preventing undigested foods and bowel toxins from escaping from the intestines into the bloodstream. During the first few weeks of an infant's life, however, the intestines allow the passage of large protein molecules through the bowel wall into the bloodstream. This is a normal and healthy situation: breast milk contains particular antibodies which need to be passed into the baby's system in order to prime the developing immune system and help to fight infection.

Because of the porous nature of babies' intestines, undigested food or bacteria can easily make their way out of the digestive tract and into the body. This makes babies prime candidates for developing food allergies and sensitivities and marks the beginning of many childhood illnesses. The porousness of babies' intestines normally changes within the first four weeks, but can take up to six months.

As a consequence, the timing of weaning, when solid foods are introduced, is very important. There is no universally correct time to introduce solid foods. A gradual introduction of new foods is the best approach. Observant parents who are aware of the potential of food allergies may be able to associate a decline in their child's health with the introduction of a particular new food.

Pregnancy

Food allergies and sensitivities have a strong hereditary association, appearing to be handed down from parent to child. The chances of a child developing sensitivities appear to be dramatically increased in cases where both parents have them.

Pregnancy is a critical time in the development of food intolerance. It is very important that allergy-prone mothers abstain from any food to which they are allergic during pregnancy so that the situation is avoided where resultant toxins reach the developing baby through the blood supply in the placenta. It is also important to try to avoid stressful situations, as tension and worry can trigger allergies.

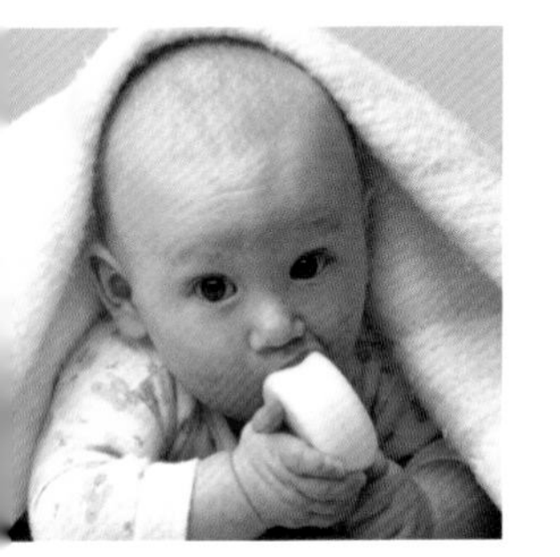

How to Assist Your Baby Further

- **Natural Birth.** Bifidobacteria and other friendly micro-organisms enter the babies' intestines as they pass through the birth canal. Babies delivered by Caesarean section have a reduced level of infiltration by these friendly micro-organisms.

- **Breast feeding.** Breast-fed babies have a lower incidence of colic and other digestive disturbances than bottle-fed babies. This is attributed to friendly bacteria (bifidobacteria), the growth of which is intensified by mother's milk. These beneficial micro-organisms account for up to 99% of healthy breast-fed babies' intestinal flora (22).

- **Long-term Feeding.** Long-term breast feeding brings added protection for the child. Feeding for less than 13 weeks results in babies suffering similar rates of intestinal problems as bottle-fed children (23).

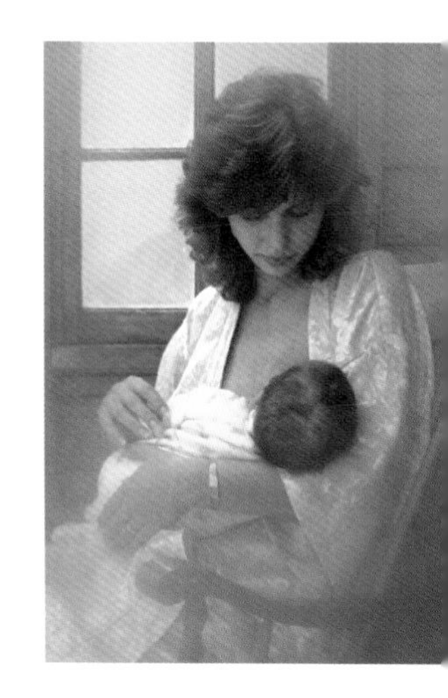

When Breast Feeding can be Problematic

The only time when breast-feeding is contra-indicated is when the mother herself has allergies. It appears that the mother's own allergy chemistry, with its associated antibodies, make their way into her milk and this upsets the child. When babies who are being breast-fed begin to develop conditions which may be allergy related, such as colic, eczema and middle ear infections, the mother should be allergy-tested first. I have observed that once a breast-feeding mother has dealt with her own allergies, her milk improves and her baby generally settles.

Conditions Affecting Babies and Children

It is my opinion that many of the common conditions of babies and children, including middle ear infections, asthma, eczema, colic and ENT problems, are strongly associated with allergies. In the majority of cases the standard treatment is either steroids or antibiotics. For most children, one short course of either does not do any particular harm. The real problems arise when the first course does not work and the child is subjected to repeat courses. Another scenario occurs when the treatment works for a short while but, within a few weeks or months, the child is ill again with the same condition. These are the circumstances in which allergy testing should definitely be considered in order to save the child from becoming debilitated from repeat courses of antibiotics and steroids.

That is, the antibiotic kills off the infection, but because the underlying cause – the allergy – is never resolved it continues to create toxins which cause further infection. As a result, the child continuously falls victim to illness. Moreover, repeated use of antibiotics or steroids disturbs the child's delicate bowel bacteria even further, and makes him or her increasingly more vulnerable to infection.

The majority of children will eventually outgrow their allergies. However, it has been my experience that the longer the undiagnosed allergy is allowed to continue and the more medication the child is given to treat the associated illnesses, the slower the child will be to outgrow the allergy.

Hyperactivity in Children

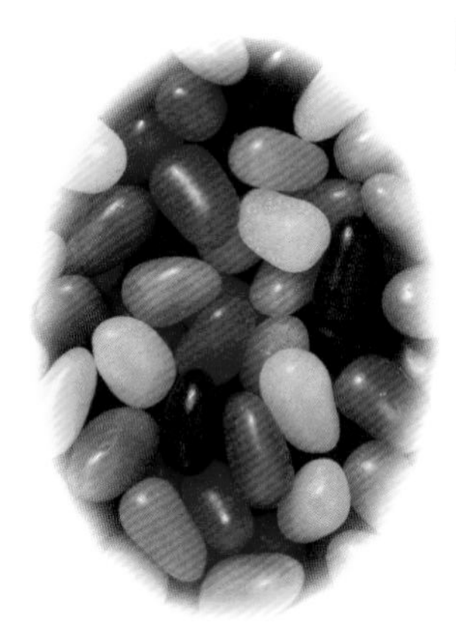

Dr. Ben Feingold was one of the first people to bring attention to the possibility of some hyperactive children being affected by food additives and colourings. However, there is also an association between hyperactivity and everyday foods such as eggs, dairy products, meat and bread. In children these reactions manifest as irritability, uncooperative behaviour and hyperactivity. In adults, such allergy reactions tend to promote mood changes, particularly depression and aggressive or anti-social impulses.

The Daily Mail *Tuesday, February 17, 1998*

Home test for foods that harm your health

By **Lesley Turney**.

Henny Hind, a mother-of-two from York, discovered allergic reactions to a multitude of common substances were at the root of her son's physical and emotional problems.

"As a toddler, Rainer suffered from recurring chest infections and severe eczema. He was hyperactive and had difficulty with sleep and concentration," says Henny, 31, who runs a health and fitness centre in York with her husband Roger.

"I was already concerned about the amount of medication he was taking and when someone suggested he might be allergic to foods I decided to have him tested.

"It transpired that Rainer was allergic, to more than 20 different foods, including wheat, oats, citrus fruits, milk and other dairy products. I removed all the allergic foods from his diet straight away.

"The eczema cleared up immediately and he had fewer and fewer infections until, a few months later, he became a perfectly healthy, happy, relaxed young boy."

(Reproduced by kind permission of The Daily Mail.)

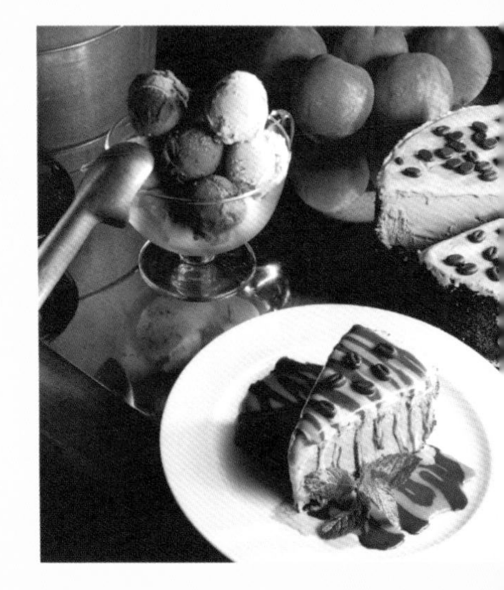

Ear Infections

Ear infections can be a complication of upper respiratory infections such as the common cold. Infection from the throat, tonsils or sinus areas can make their way into the middle ear through the Eustachian tube, although normally the design of the tube prevents this from happening.

Other middle ear infections, common in babies and children, have a strong allergy association. One such condition is otitis media. The middle ear is connected to the throat by the Eustachian tube, which drains the fluids that occur naturally within the middle ear. The Eustachian tube can become inflamed, swollen, and ultimately blocked. When this happens, fluid builds up behind the ear drum and creates pressure in the middle ear. The fluid can then become stagnant and infected. The pressure alone is a source of great discomfort for affected children, and infected fluid leads to inflammation of the ear drum and surrounding tissues.

The child may cry persistently, rub the ear, have a fever, be irritable and may have difficulty in hearing. Symptoms associated with middle ear infection also include diarrhoea and vomiting.

The standard treatment for ear infections is to prescribe antibiotics. Children are often given repeat courses of antibiotics for recurring infections. This means, however, that these children build up resistance and, as a consequence, require stronger antibiotics. Some doctors prescribe antibiotics to be taken daily to prevent ear infection in those who are prone to such infections. Sometimes an operation is performed to insert a tube (grommet) to drain the fluid from the ear.

And yet, children who are tested for food sensitivities can potentially be spared this medication and surgery.

Leeds Weekly News *Thursday, July 22, 1999*

Twins Maria and Jenny Harnett (names changed), who doctors discovered have an allergy to dairy products

By **Sheila Holmes**.

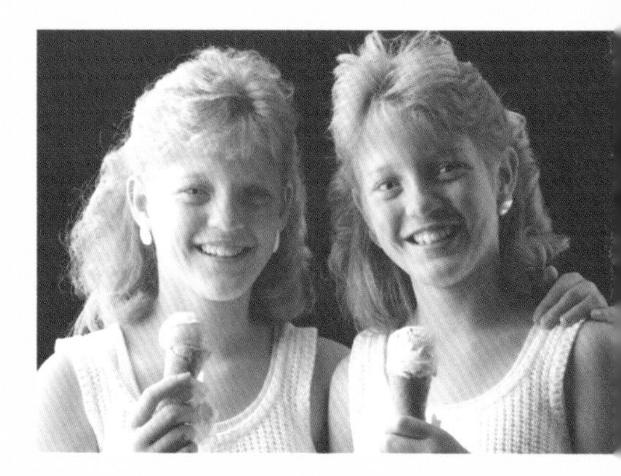

Since they were a week old, identical Leeds twins Maria and Jenny Harnett have been plagued with persistent ear infections. Their mum Deborah has taken the girls back and forth to the doctor, the paediatrician and the hospital for the past six years.

But despite having five operations to insert grommets to try to stop their constant pain, the twins did not grow out of the problem as promised, their hearing deteriorated and their temperaments worsened.

Finally Deborah decided to take them for a food sensitivity test (...). It was discovered that the twins had identical severe sensitivities to egg white and cow's milk and sensitivities to goat's milk, almonds and cola.

And just 10 days after changing their diet, Deborah could see noticeable improvement in the health of both the girls. She said: "Ever since they were babies the girls would cry and scream at night and were very unsettled.

"It was extremely worrying to watch the girls go through the operations at such a young age.

"Both Maria and Jenny have had far more antibiotics than the average child has. I knew that something must be causing their infections, but I could not pinpoint what it was.

"Now they are more confident and much happier. Overall they look healthier, they behave much better and I can only assume that this is because they feel so much better."

Both girls, who had not put on weight for a number of months, have now reached their correct weight, their hearing has improved, the ear infections have gone, the congestion in their sinuses has gone and they have stopped snoring at night.

(Leeds Weekly News, Thursday, July 22, 1999.)

Chapter Seven

Some Common Conditions

(and how to help them)

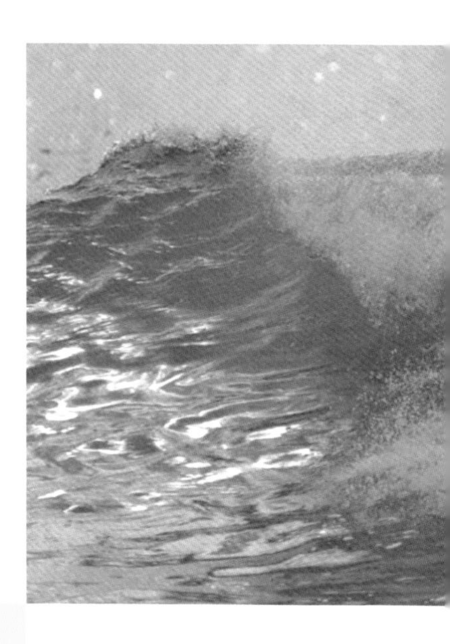

A short book of this kind cannot possibly detail how to deal with every allergy-related illness. Perhaps it does not need to, since I believe that many common medical conditions are but different manifestations of the same phenomenon – allergy. The treatment approach which I have found to be most effective in these associated conditions is allergy testing, dietary change and acupuncture. Although the basic principles are the same, to get the very best results the treatment should be tailored to the individual's needs.

Throughout this book there are examples of allergy-related illnesses and case histories showing how disruptive and distressing symptoms were alleviated by tracing them back to the source. This chapter deals with a further three common conditions:

- irritable bowel syndrome (IBS);
- migraine;
- stomach ulcers.

Irritable Bowel Syndrome (IBS)

According to a survey conducted in 1998 for the anti-spasmodic drug Colpermin, one in five adults suffers the symptoms of irritable bowel syndrome (IBS), a disturbance of normal bowel function which manifests as abdominal discomfort and difficult or uncomfortable bowel habits. IBS is far more common in women, with 28% suffering symptoms, compared to 11% of men. In Ireland today it is a strikingly common condition. According to Dr. N. Keeling (St. James Hospital, Dublin), a specialist in bowel disorders IBS affects about 15 out of every 16 patients who attend his hospital gastroenterology clinic (24).

The word "irritable" refers to the fact that the nerve endings supplying the bowel are very sensitive. As a result the bowel becomes irritated by the slightest disturbance from food particles, fluids or gas passing along its length. Symptoms commonly include one or all of the following:

- Intestinal spasm, cramps and abdominal discomfort;
- Bloating, flatulence, nausea;
- Constipation and/or diarrhoea;
- Incomplete bowel movements.

IBS presents no evidence of actual disease in the bowel itself. Diagnosis is often made on the basis of the above symptoms together with the absence of evidence of any organic disease. Blood tests, X-rays and endoscopy are sometimes used to confirm diagnosis. However, as bowel cancer could be a possibility, a proper diagnosis must always first be obtained before the allergy approach is investigated.

In my mind there is little doubt that IBS is brought about by emotional stress, tension being relayed to the bowel through the nerve pathways to make it abnormally sensitive. The sensitivity of the bowel reflects the degree of stress experienced. Undigested foods then further aggravate an already sensitive bowel and act as the trigger that initiates the symptoms.

The Sunday Telegraph *March 21, 1999*

Revealed: the healthy foods that make you ill

By **Jacqui Thornton**

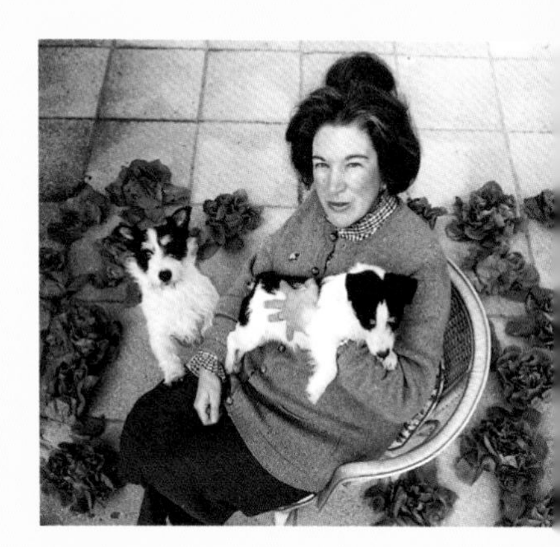

For years, parents have been telling children to eat their greens and fill up with fruit to keep healthy. But new research shows that some of the vegetables, beans and fruit that we have been encouraged to eat are likely to make us ill. (...)

Scientists have discovered that blackcurrants, kidney beans, tomatoes, peas and even lettuce can all have adverse effects. (...)

The foods themselves do not cause the symptoms but, rather, trigger an adverse reaction in people with a disposition to those symptoms. Thus someone disposed to migraine will suffer bad headaches if they eat the food to which they are sensitive. (...)

Tony Robards, professor of biology and pro-vice-chancellor of the University of York, (...) said: "Who would believe that the friendly old lettuce would make someone feel very unwell? But if it's got a certain molecule in it your body may not like it."

He said that food sensitivity was triggered by the rejection of an ingested substance by the body's immune system. "The human body has developed a sophisticated defence against being attacked on all sides. When it sees something it does not like it produces an allergic response." He said this could be extreme and immediate, as with shellfish, or a less evident reaction that could be measured in antibodies in the blood. (...)

Christine Alden was cured of her ills after cutting out lettuce and fruit.

Christine, 44, a farmer's wife (...), was amazed to discover that she was sensitive to lettuce, grapefruit, pineapple and cola drinks. She had long suffered from irritable bowel syndrome and had tried to eat healthily as a result.

She was on prescription drugs but felt depressed and lethargic and had stomach pain. After taking the test she lost a stone and dispensed with her drugs. "I couldn't believe it. I switched to lettuce and fruit juice because I thought they were healthy".

Migraine

A migraine is a recurring, throbbing headache. Migraines are believed to be the end result of blood vessels in the brain becoming distended and inflamed. Sometimes this period of inflammation is followed by a constriction of the blood vessels.

There is often a warning (aura) of an approaching attack. This ranges from visual disturbance such as bright spots and zigzag lines, to tingling or weakness in the limbs or drowsiness. Not everyone experiences this aura, but when a person does, symptoms tend to occur in the same combination in each attack. These are called classic migraines. Another type, known as common migraine, shows without warning.

Just as the bowel has a direct nerve supply, there is also a nerve supply to the blood vessels, controlling their dilation and constriction. In times of emergency this nerve supply constricts the diameter of the blood vessels, increasing the pressure and improving blood supply throughout the entire body. Once the emergency has passed they release the constriction and the pressure lessens.

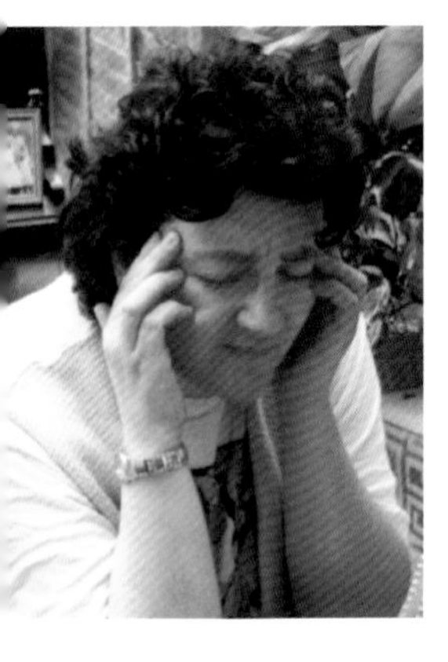

These nerve pathways can become overcharged when the individual is under stress causing blood vessels to over-constrict or over-dilate, and may become inflamed. Toxins from undigested foods target the already inflamed blood vessels and aggravate the symptoms of the migraine.

The Daily Express *Friday, June 30, 2000*

Muesli made me sneeze for 35 years

By **Alun Rees**

Allergy victim Patrick Webster sneezed 700 times a day for 35 years until specialists discovered his nightmare affliction was caused by the "healthy" bowl of muesli he ate every morning.

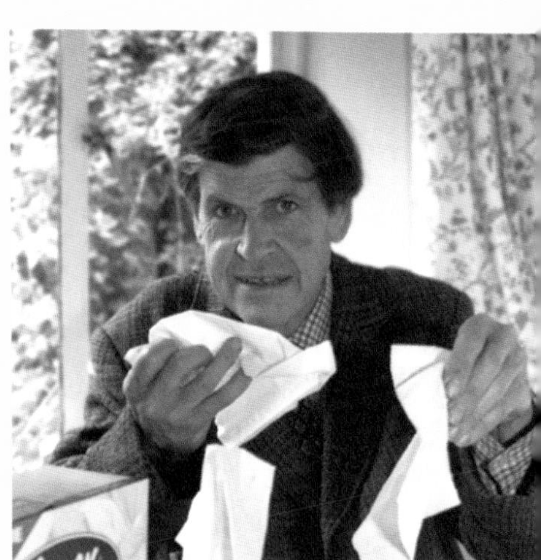

The 52-year-old former civil servant had gone to more than 60 NHS doctors in his quest for relief but the sneezing went on and on until last July he went private and visited an allergy clinic two hundred miles from home.

Now Patrick is considering legal action against his health authority, claiming their inability to spot his allergy to oats and egg yolk through a series of food sensitivity elimination tests amounts to negligence.

Patrick, whose attacks began at 15, said: "I sneezed hundreds of times a day, all year round and it was exhausting. I was so desperate to try to sort it out that I took six months off work and ended up in three different hospitals. I had skin tests for allergies but they were negative so the doctors would not give me any other sort of allergy tests.

"One doctor even told me I must be allergic to myself, so it is no wonder I did not get any better. The best treatment they could offer me was steroids and for 20 years I practically lived on them but it was an utter waste of time and did more harm than good.

"Now I do not need them but I am left with all the side effects like osteoporosis, cramp and a very low mineral count."

Stomach Ulcers

The term refers to an area of erosion or inflammation of the mucous membrane lining of the stomach. The usual symptoms are pain in this general area, accompanied by vomiting, heartburn or flatulence. Attacks may last for several weeks and then clear up completely, only to recur again unexpectedly.

In investigating the cause of stomach ulcers, interest recently has centred on helicobacter pylori (HP), a stomach bacterium. A combination of three very powerful antibiotics are currently used to eradicate this organism.

Half of the world's population is thought to be infected with HP. Given that the gastrointestinal tract is normally inhabited by more than two-and-a-half pounds of live bacteria, HP may well be a natural intestinal bacterium which has increased in numbers. But if HP is the cause of gastric ulcers, why is it that the half of the world's population, who are also infected with HP, do not suffer from ulcers?

The HP hypothesis appears to me to be very similar to the explanation of candida discussed in Chapter 5 above. My view is that all of these potentially harmful bacteria can be kept in check only by a strong immune system and by flourishing populations of healthy bacteria.

In some cases antibiotics resolve the problem but for many it is only a matter of time before the condition reappears. In such cases the conventional medical approach is to use an even stronger course of antibiotics. The end result is that the patient becomes seriously depleted from these powerful drugs.

CHAPTER EIGHT

Hormones and HRT

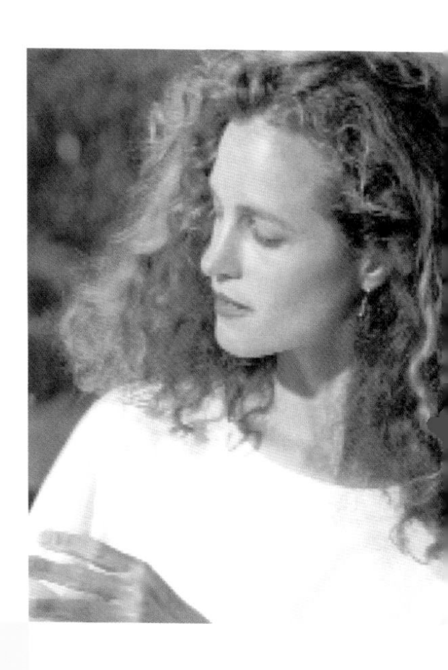

Hormones are chemical messengers which travel throughout the body in the bloodstream. They influence the performance of many of the body's most important organs and body systems.

Hormone Replacement Therapy (HRT) consists of specific hormones, usually taken orally, by women who are thought to be suffering from hormonal deficiencies.

There are a number of medical problems specific to women, notably osteoporosis and hot flushes, which are associated with degrees of imbalance within the female hormonal system. Western medicine tends to believe that HRT is the solution to the majority of these problems.

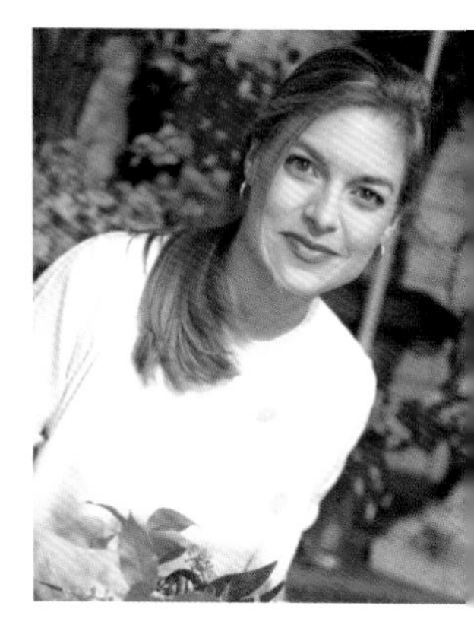

Women who are prone to allergies often respond very badly to HRT. They can feel marvellous for the first six months to two years, but then the side-effects begin. Because of this delayed reaction, these side-effects, such as allergies, weight gain, bloating and generally feeling unwell, are not recognised as being caused by HRT.

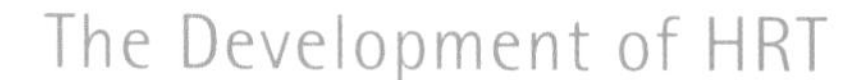

The Development of HRT

Oestrogen preparations became available in the 1920s and have since had a chequered history. In the 1960s it was believed they were a wonder drug, able to cure many of the disorders of mid-life, and with the potential to delay the onset of aging. However, in the mid 1970s it was discovered that the use of oestrogen caused a marked increase in the incidence of endometrial cancer (cancer of the lining of the womb). HRT has been re-formulated and re-launched with the addition of progesterone, which is now believed to protect the endometrium from cancer. However, there are many continuing doubts about its safety (25).

A Mistaken Theory

The female hormones, oestrogen and progesterone, work together as a pair. Oestrogen stimulates many of the female body systems and progesterone protects these systems from over-stimulation. In particular, oestrogen stimulates breast and uterine lining.

Doctors believe that many of the female complaints associated with the menopause are caused by oestrogen deficiency, and that conditions such as osteoporosis, heart disease and hot flushing can be resolved by HRT. However, I have become increasingly alarmed at the number of female allergy patients whose lives were being made very much worse by HRT. I was shocked to find that there is very scant evidence to support many of the supposed benefits of HRT, and in fact volumes of evidence warning of the dangers involved (25a).

The majority of women are rarely, if ever, tested to assess their exact hormone levels before HRT is prescribed. It is instead prescribed in standard doses and its appropriateness assessed on whether it causes side-effects or not. Side-effects, however, can take between six months and two years to appear and, because of the time delay, are not then associated with the HRT.

Hormone Tests

The FSH/LH Test

There are several tests available to doctors wishing to measure hormone levels. The Follicle-Stimulating Hormone/Luteinizing Hormone (FSH/LH) Test is the most common, but it is unsatisfactory because it does not measure your actual working oestrogen and progesterone hormone levels directly. Instead, it measures FSH and LH levels – hormones sent out by the brain to trigger production of oestrogen and progesterone. The practitioner then has to interpret the significance of these readings and they are easily misinterpreted.

Blood Tests

Blood tests are used to measure hormone levels, but these also have disadvantages. Of the total number of hormones in your bloodstream, only a very small number of free hormones, between 1% and 10%, are of benefit to the body at any given time. The majority are in a form that the body cannot use (bound hormones). Blood tests record your overall hormone levels but are unable to advise how much of that is of any use to you. Given that some of these hormones are measured in one-billionth of a gram (equivalent to a pinch of salt in a swimming-pool), you can see how precise a hormone test really needs to be.

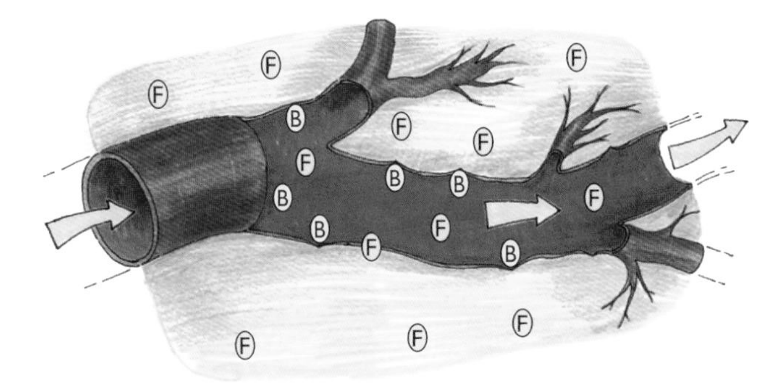

Ⓕ Free unbound hormones

Ⓑ Bound hormones

Saliva Tests

There is a much better way of testing for oestrogen and progesterone hormone levels. Only those hormones that can breakout and penetrate the tissues are of any real use to you. These free, unbound hormones also enter into your saliva and can easily be measured there.

A major advantage of the saliva test has to do with the time of day the sample is collected. Hormone levels rise and fall throughout the day, and it is best to collect the sample at the same time each day. Blood tests can only be taken at hospitals, clinics or GP surgeries, and it is therefore more difficult to collect a blood sample at consistent times.

Saliva testing is done in the privacy of your own home. A small saliva sample is collected in a special container and this is then posted to the laboratory for analysis. An early morning sample, before eating or brushing your teeth, is recommended.

Saliva testing has been used scientifically for about thirty years. However, it has been used primarily in research institutes and as a consequence remains an unfamiliar technique to many practitioners.

Hormone Types

Not only are women receiving the incorrect dosage of hormones but they are also receiving the wrong type of hormones.

Hormones come in three types: natural, synthetic and animal-derived. Natural hormones are the same as your own and work in exactly the same way. These natural hormones are of plant origin, but still have to be processed by a laboratory. They are sometimes known as bio-identical hormones and are processed in such a way that they remain an identical match with your own.

However, the most commonly prescribed hormones are either synthetic or animal-derived. The pharmaceutical companies promote these synthetic hormones because they are the only ones they can patent. Synthetic and animal-derived hormones are similar to your own, but they are not an exact match. In fact these synthetic and animal-derived hormones can actually aggravate many hormone associated symptoms (25a), such as:

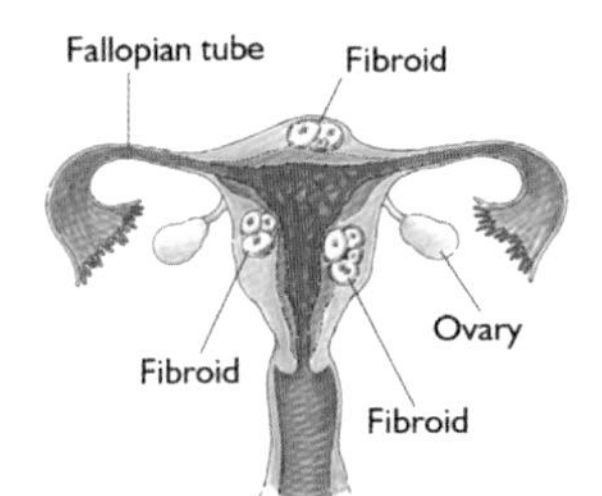

- Fibroids;
- Weight gain, bloating, swollen, tender breasts;
- Increased blood pressure;
- Irritability, depression, hot flushes, night sweats;

- Exacerbation of allergy symptoms such as asthma, eczema, migraine, irritable bowel, arthritis.

Another problem with these poorly fitting hormones is that the body has great difficulty in excreting them. Natural hormones are excreted from the body within hours, but some of these artificial hormones have been shown to remain within the body for up to thirteen weeks. Therefore many of the side-effects are the result of hormonal over-stimulation.

Natural Progesterone

Menopausal decrease in oestrogen is estimated to be approximately 60%, whereas progesterone depletion can be 100%. As a result of this new understanding of hormonal levels, many practitioners are now not prescribing HRT but instead are prescribing natural progesterone. Natural progesterone on its own, without the problematic oestrogen, is proving to be a useful, apparently side-effect free method of treating many of the hormone-related conditions previously treated with HRT. A general misconception is that natural progesterone and the synthetic forms (known as progestins or progestogens) are much the same thing. They are not. An increasing body of evidence (25c) indicates that synthetic progestins do not work as well as natural progesterone and have many toxic side-effects.

At the present time natural progesterone is undergoing major clinical trials, and many more still need to be conducted. All the evidence so far, including that of a lifetime's study by Dr. J. Lee, indicate that when taken in the correct dosage, natural progesterone is side-effect free.

In some countries natural progesterone is available at your local pharmacy without prescription; in other countries it is prescription only. Enquire from your own practitioner or local pharmacy.

Hormone Replacement Therapy (HRT)

Hormone replacement comes in a variety of forms and three of the most popular are tablets, patches or creams.

Hormones in tablet form have to pass through your digestive system and your liver, so only about 10% of the original dose finally makes its way into your bloodstream to work for you. Because of this, the prescribed dosage is very high, and this causes many of the side-effects which are so commonly associated with the tablet form.

The patch is a small hormone reservoir which is attached to the skin with a sticking plaster and is changed once or twice a week. The hormones pass directly into your bloodstream, and the dosage is considerably lower than tablets, sometimes as much as ten times lower. Most patches come only in standard doses, so it is more difficult to adjust the dosage.

Natural progesterone creams are impregnated with hormone and then absorbed directly through the skin. As with the patch, therapeutic results are achieved through relatively low dosages. The great advantage of creams is that the dosage can easily be adjusted by the individual.

Osteoporosis

The average woman has achieved maximum bone strength by the age of 25 to 35, after which it begins slowly to leak away. Osteoporosis means literally "porous bones". It is a disease in which the bones become very porous, increasingly fragile, and prone to easily breaking. It shows no outward signs, however, until it is firmly established. Osteoporosis can affect the whole skeleton but more commonly causes vulnerability to fracture in spine, hip and wrist bones.

The medical establishment believes that oestrogen deficiency is the primary cause of this condition, and that HRT is the treatment of choice. The reality is that osteoporosis is a disease of excessive bone loss, but not necessarily because of oestrogen deficiency.

Many women suffering with osteoporosis arrive at menopause with the condition well established. It may have started many years beforehand, when oestrogen levels are often at their highest. Once menopause begins, these women then experience an increase in the rate of loss of bone mineral density which is more than the average rate of loss. This accelerated loss continues for a period of about five years. During this period HRT temporarily curtails the rate of loss of bone mass, but it does not significantly build new bone tissue (25d).

Any benefits associated with HRT are lost within five to ten years. Thus these women arrive in their seventies, which is the most vulnerable time for fractures, without any protection (as they would have done without HRT).

The new and better saliva tests indicate in these cases that oestrogen is deficient, but very often it is the progesterone that is even more deficient. Dr. Lee's research has shown that women will gain new bone, of a higher bone-mineral density, from natural progesterone therapy, with or without the problematic oestrogen (25e). The hugely important PEPI trial in 1995 (25f) proved that natural progesterone was superior to synthetic.

Four Key Factors in the Prevention of Osteoporosis

- The first cause of osteoporosis is a Hormonal imbalance, especially between oestrogen and progesterone. If you do decide to use hormones to help this situation, you must first of all have your levels tested. Only use natural hormones, and check your levels at regular intervals to ensure you are not overdosing your system.
- Calcium is a major component of the building blocks of bone. Dairy products are the number one source of calcium for the

majority of people; yet allergies to dairy products are almost endemic to Western societies. If you are allergic to dairy products you will extract no calcium from them. The IgG allergy test is the only way to be certain whether you are allergic to dairy products or not.

- Regular exercise is an essential factor in maintaining good general health; but it is especially important for maintaining healthy bone structure.

- Stress is the vital ingredient in all of the conditions mentioned in this book. Stress knocks the entire hormonal orchestra out of balance and in my view is the initiator of the entire condition. A regular exercise programme, especially if it is exercise that you enjoy, is one of the best and most natural ways of dealing with general lifestyle stress.

The other treatment option is to use Five Element Acupuncture. It requires great skill on the part of a practitioner but I regard acupuncture as one of the most under-rated, yet most powerful, ways to rebalance your entire hormonal system.

A Recommended Test for Osteoporosis

Healthy vertebra

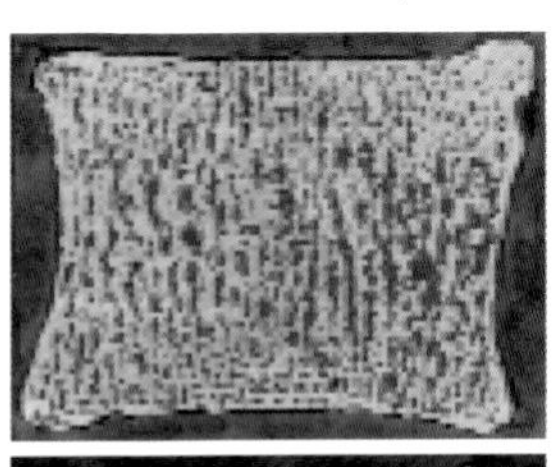

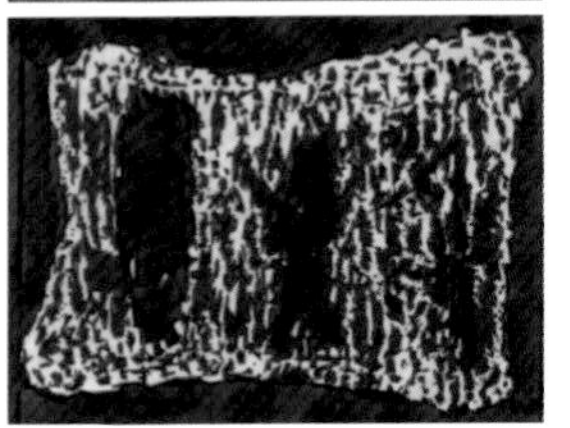

Osteoporosis of vertebra

Osteoporosis gives few warning signals. It often takes a sudden or unexpected fracture to highlight the reality that the condition is well established. Once bone density has been severely lost, it is very difficult to re-establish the same bone strength. So it is vital to diagnose this condition as early as possible.

If you are diagnosed with osteoporosis you will need to begin a course of treatment immediately. You may decide to use HRT, or you may decide to use a more natural approach such as acupuncture, natural progesterone, calcium supplements, and exercise. Once you begin treatment you will then need to know if the treatment is working. The only way of confirming this is to have a diagnostic test. There are several tests available, and they use a variety of ultrasound and X-ray techniques to assess your bone density. Measurements are taken every two or three years so as to track your progress.

X-ray tests tell you what has happened to your bones, giving your present density levels. However, the loss may have occurred many years earlier during a period of particular ill-health and have now stopped. Or it may have happened around the time of menopause but have since stopped. In short, X-rays can only tell you what has happened, not what is happening right now.

A better test is available, known as The Deoxypyridinoline Test (Dpd). It tells you what is happening to your bones on any given day, and whether the accelerated bone loss you suffered at some stage in your life has now stopped. Equally it can tell you if the bone loss is continuing and if so, whether it is at a very slow or at an alarming rate. If you begin a course of treatment, it will tell you within weeks if the treatment is helping your condition.

The Dpd Test measures the level of a substance known as Dpd, which is released during the breakdown of bone cells and is excreted from the body in urine. It is a very specific marker of bone disintegration and one which the laboratory can measure. All you have to do is collect your first morning urine sample in a special container and post it to one of the laboratories.

Conclusion

The scientific community is convinced of the enormous potential of Hormone Replace Therapy. HRT has indeed a great potential, but not as it is at present being practised, not by using artificial hormones, and certainly not by prescribing them without first testing existing hormone levels to prevent overdosing.

What is very clear to me is that a considerable number of women are being made very much worse by HRT. The side-effects take a long time to develop and because of this they are often not associated with HRT.

The scientific community's unshakable belief in HRT is based upon scant endorsements of something with potentially serious side-effects. Leaving aside all the supposed science associated with this, common sense tells us that something which is supposed to cure you should certainly not also predispose you to the risk of further serious illness.

It is my view that there are important and better options available, and this book is intended throughout to inform you of your options. Furthermore, in my view, there is a broad group of symptoms which are thought to be hormonal, but which are in fact allergic reactions.

However, this book is certainly not intended as a replacement for a competent practitioner who is familiar with the new tests, and could guide you safely through this maze of information.

The Sunday Times *April 9, 2000*

Stroke risk for 1.3 HRT women

By **Jonathan Leake** *and* **Sophie Petit-Zeman**.

Millions of women taking hormone replacement therapy could be running an increased risk of heart attacks and strokes, research has shown. The study of 25,000 women in America has caused consternation among researchers who had expected to find that women taking HRT stood less chance of such attacks.

It comes just two years into a 10-year study and has forced the researchers, along with the doctors conducting a similar trial in Britain, to write to all the women involved warning them that they could be at risk. (...)

Professor Marcia Stefanick, a researcher at Stanford Medical Centre in California who is leading a large part of the American government-funded study, confirmed that there has been "an increase in cardiovascular events" but added that the findings were preliminary and should be treated with caution. However, she added: "This highlights how little we know about a subject people think we know so much about."

Case History

Dolores Melinn*, Dublin, Ireland.

Dolores has been on and off HRT for the past six years. It was prescribed as a result of osteoporosis and other hormone related problems (hot flushes, poor concentration, general hormonal symptoms), all of which left her feeling physically and emotionally drained.

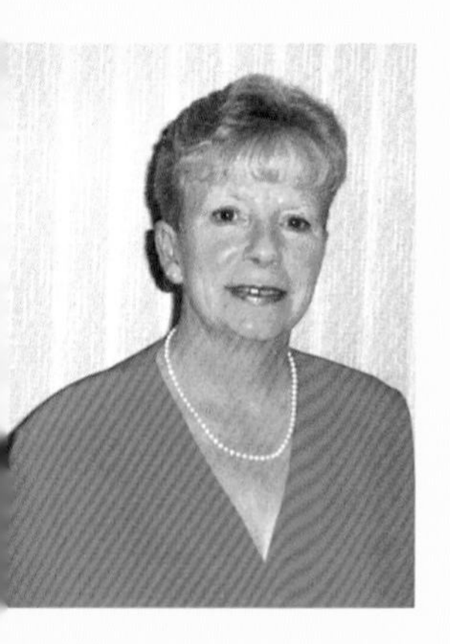

She had her last period in June 1994, after which many of the problems began. She started HRT in March 1995 and felt very much better for about six months. Then everything began to go wrong. She developed chronic back pain with a gross swelling at the top of her spine. Eventually she stopped HRT herself because the back pain was terrible and within a short time of stopping, the back and neck improved.

One year later, as a result of the progression of the osteoporosis, Dolores broke a bone in her foot and was put back on HRT. Again within about six months all of the terrible back and neck pains had returned. She was referred to a consultant who told her to stay on HRT as it was not connected with her back pains. Eventually the back and neck pains got to the point of being unbearable and she stopped HRT herself. Within days of stopping HRT all of these intractable pains were considerably improved. However, all the hot flushes and other hormone related problems returned.

Throughout all of this, Dolores has never had her hormone levels tested. I did the saliva test for her and the results came back showing an excess of oestrogen within her system. Therefore, her bad reaction to HRT was most likely due to an overdose of hormones.

Dolores had the IgG allergy test and was found to be highly allergic. A prescribed change of diet brought about a remarkable, 80% improvement in her general health. She started taking a regular calcium supplement. A course of acupuncture greatly assisted in stabilizing the hormonal balance.

The most recent Dpd osteoporosis assessment test indicates that Dolores' osteoporosis has stopped progressing. She has returned to full health without HRT.

* A patient of the author.

Chapter Nine

Allergy Tests

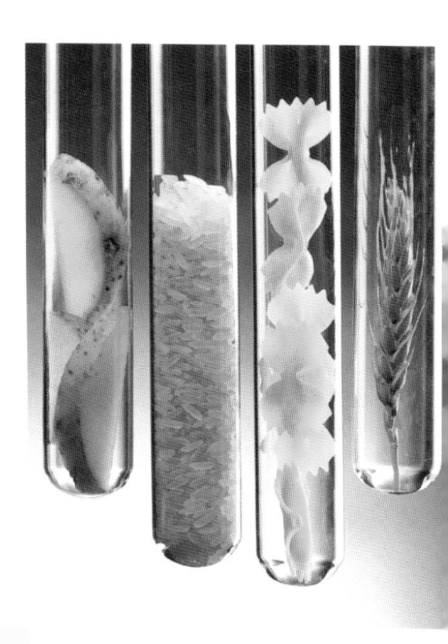

This book has so far argued that unfriendly bacteria which produce specific toxins are stimulated by certain foods, medications and by worry and stress. This situation is exacerbated when allergic foods (undigested foods) arrive in the intestines and interact with these unfriendly bacteria, leading to an escalation of toxicity in the bowel. Allergy testing is about identifying those foods which are responsible for this escalation of toxicity, with a view to removing them from the diet. This results in a rapid and dramatic improvement in health. The two situations in which the removal of the allergy foods alone may not improve the situation are:

- Allergic reaction to medication, where the person nevertheless continues to take the offending drug.
- A person failing to reduce stress and tension in his or her life.

There are many kinds of allergy testing available. For an allergy testing approach to be viable and useful it should fulfil certain criteria:

- The test must be objective, not subject to human interpretation as this can lead to results which are influenced by the tester's own bias or beliefs.
- The test must be reproducible: if a person's test substance (blood) is submitted several times, it should give the same result each time.
- The test must be able to grade the degree of allergy reaction. People who have food allergies generally have two or three primary allergies, along with a small number of secondary allergies. It has been my experience that the avoidance of the primary allergies alone is generally sufficient to resolve the problem. Tests which are unable to grade the degree of allergy reaction result in patients having to avoid all kinds of foods, which is both difficult and inconvenient. Ultimately people are unlikely to stick to strict regimes which exclude too many foods.

Many of the tests currently available are relevant for detecting classic IgE fast-reacting allergies, whereas **the majority of food allergies are primarily slow-reacting and triggered by IgG antibodies.**

I am at present using a specific IgG test which satisfies all of the above criteria.

The IgG Test and How it Works

As already noted, it is only in the past five years that American researchers have come to understand the IgG antibody. Since then a diagnostic test has been developed to assist in pinpointing slow-response food allergies. Trials have been conducted which endorse the IgG test (26), and others are underway. Having been involved with allergy testing since 1983, and having worked with nearly every test available, I am in no doubt that the IgG test is the best and most useful tool currently available (27).

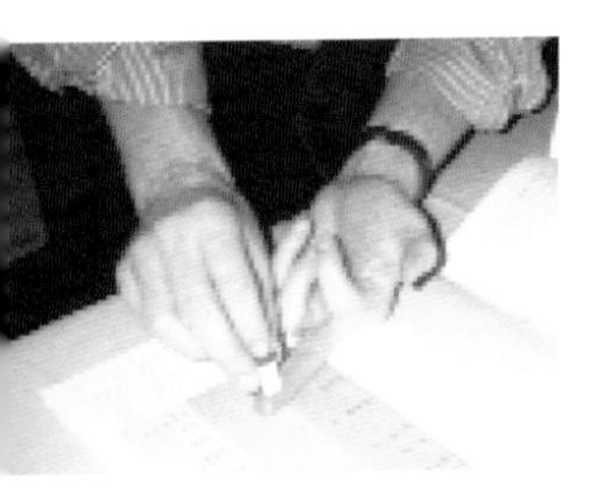

In addition to an excellent record of reproducibility, the IgG test used by my clinic is able to grade the degree of reaction of the specific food and is not subject to human interpretation. The other great advantage of the test is that it can be conducted in the person's own home. Only a pinprick drop of blood is required, just like that used by diabetics to check their blood sugar levels. The patient is supplied with an easy-to-use extractor kit with full instructions. The drop of blood is returned in a specially prepared container and is then analysed at the laboratory.

The laboratory analysis uses specially designed test plates which have small wells on the surface. Foods considered most likely to cause allergic responses are cultured in the wells, and the patient's blood is spread across the plate. If the blood contains antibodies which are antagonistic to a particular food, they will attach themselves to the inside of that well. After a set period of time, the plate is washed clean of all remaining blood particles so that only the attached antibodies remain. A special coloured dye is then added which binds with the attached test-antibodies on the plate. The deeper the resulting colour,

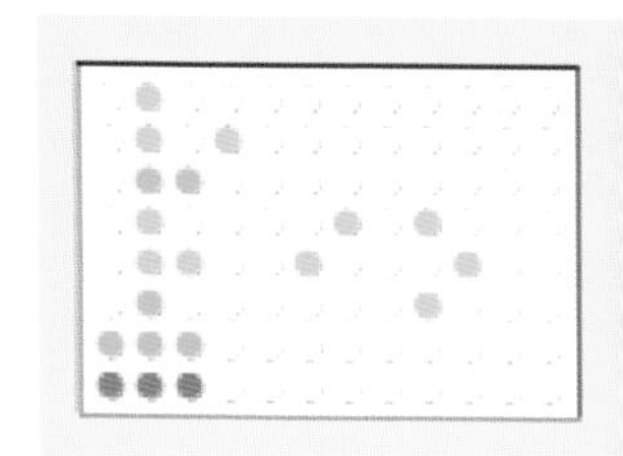

the greater the amount of food-specific antibody present in any particular test plate well. By using sophisticated instrumentation which can interpret the depth of colour, it is possible to measure the precise antibody level.

It is important to note that the test only works on foods which have been consumed within a period of three months prior to taking the blood sample, so it is important to eat a good cross-section of foods, especially the foods which you specifically want to have investigated, before taking the test.

Interpreting the Test Results

On completion of the laboratory analysis, a result sheet grading (see p 81) the level of allergy reaction to each food tested is returned to the client. Accurate interpretation of this information is vital if people are to achieve the maximum benefit from the test.

This test grades reactions into three basic categories according to the amount of food-specific antibody detected.

"Avoid", "Rotate" and "No Reaction".

The "Avoid" group is further categorized into +1, +2, +3 and +4, according to the degree of severity of the reaction, +4 being the most serious.

How to Start Your Diet

Avoid These are your primary allergies. Eliminate these foods from your diet completely. You will need to avoid these for three months minimum.

Rotate These are your secondary allergies. Eliminate these for a period of four weeks. After that you should be much improved and you can begin to reintroduce these foods one at a time. Leave at least two days between each food. If the reintroduced food leads to a return of the symptoms you can be certain which food is responsible.

No Reaction You can eat these foods as normal.

Test Results

In general the severity of the reaction as indicated on the test result sheet correlates with the severity of the symptoms caused by the food in question. For example, the Yeast +3 reaction shown is to be suspected to be the primary culprit. In the majority of cases you can be certain that a high reading in the "Avoid" column is the main instigator of your distress and should be the food that receives your closest attention. However, in a small number of cases, the food listed in the "Rotate" column will also be actively involved in keeping the disease process active. I advocate a four week elimination procedure to verify the results.

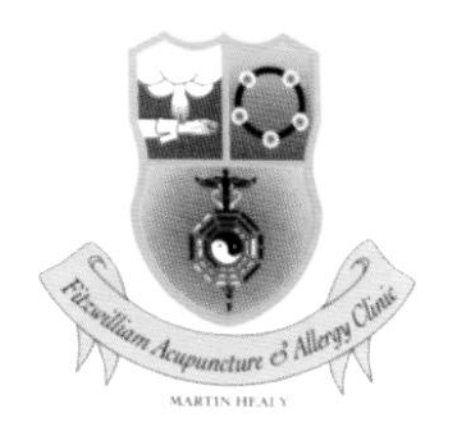

	AVOID	ROTATE	NO REACTION
Grains			Wheat
		Oat	
			Rice
			Rye
			Corn
Dairy			Cows Milk
		Egg White	
			Egg Yolk
Fish			White Fish Mix
	Shellfish Mix +1		
Vegetables			Carrot
			Legume Mix
			Mustard Mix
		Potato	
Fruits			Apple/Pear
			Berry Mix
			Citrus Mix
Nuts			Nut Mix
Others	Yeast +3		
Meats			Chicken/Turkey
			Pork

INDIVIDUAL COMPONENTS OF FOOD MIXES

White Fish Mix	Shellfish Mix	Legume Mix	Mustard Mix
Cod	Crab	Haricot Bean	Cabbage
Haddock	Lobster	Kidney Bean	Broccoli
Plaice	Prawn	Soya Bean	Cauliflower
		Pea	

Berry Mix	Citrus Mix	Nut mix	Yeast
Raspberry	Orange	Almond	Yeast Bakers
Strawberry	Lemon	Cashew	Yeast Brewers
Blackberry	Grapefruit	Hazelnut	
		Peanut	

Note: The results of this test must be brought to the attention of your GP as he may wish to adjust his treatment plan or any medication you are taking.

Other Allergy Tests

In my view the IgG test is the best available for identifying slow-response food allergies. There are, however, many others currently available, and their advantages and disadvantages are discussed below.

The Prick & Scratch Method

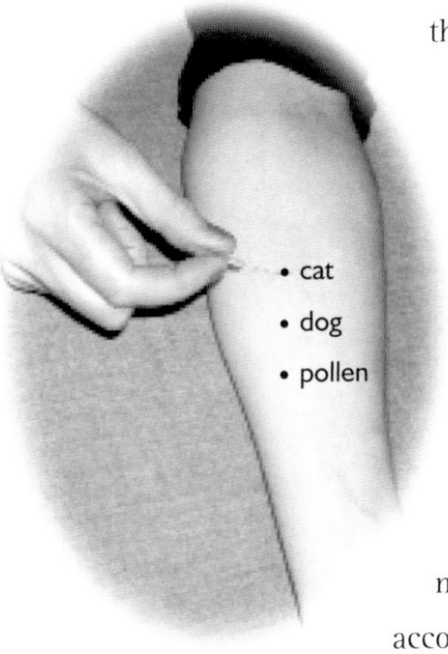

The first allergy test to be used by Western medical practitioners was the prick and scratch method. This is still the standard hospital test today. It was introduced around 1911 and has not developed much since then. A small drop of the test substance is dropped onto the skin, which is then either scratched or pricked with a needle. The amount of inflammation which develops at the scratch site indicates how allergic to the substance the subject is. Applied to detect an adverse reaction to food, however, the test merely determines whether a crude food extract can provoke the release of histamine from skin mast cells. In reality the majority of clinical symptoms triggered by food allergies are not mediated by this mechanism of response (28). This test is accordingly inaccurate when applied for the detection of the majority of food allergies and intolerances: it gives many false readings. Skin prick tests have been shown to produce positive readings in the cases of only 15% of known food sensitivities. Furthermore, about 60% of foods which test positive by this test have no effect upon the individual concerned (29). The prick and scratch method appears to work better when testing for external factors, such as dust and animal hairs, and for IgE reactions.

Patch Testing

A similar technique used in hospitals is patch testing. Small quantities of suspected substances are placed under individual cups which are then taped to the skin for a number of hours. A reddening of the skin under the patch denotes a sensitivity to that particular substance. As with the prick and scratch method, patch testing is perhaps more appropriate for testing external agents but almost of no value for checking for food allergies. Foods and other substances which are well-known by the individual to cause clearly identifiable reactions commonly fail to react with this test.

Cytotoxic Testing

This is a laboratory test using the subject's blood in which the white blood cells are separated by centrifuge. These are then placed on a slide and the foods to be tested are added. A laboratory technician records the effects on the blood cells. The dependence on human interpretation is a major weakness, especially when multiple samples have to be monitored. The test was first introduced into the UK in the 1950s with a claim of 80% accuracy. It is currently in disrepute because of an inability to duplicate the findings from one laboratory to another, or even within the same laboratory on different runs (30).

The RAST Test

The RAST Test (radioimmunoassay) is another allergy test using blood. It is designed to detect the presence of IgE. However, in the case of foods, the value of the RAST test is limited, not because of its in-accuracy but because it measures only IgE, which accounts for only a small proportion of the food hypersensitivities (31).

The Elimination Diet

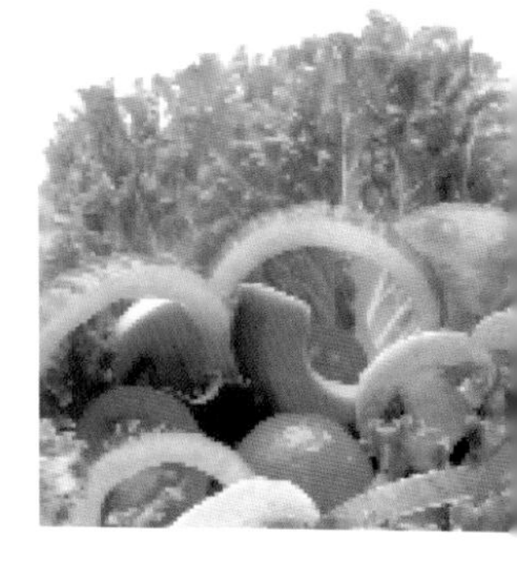

By the mid 1960s the existence of slow-response food allergies had begun to emerge, but without there being any reliable scientific method to identify them. As a result there was a lot of interest in "trial and error" styles of testing. The best known of these is the Elimination Diet, also known as the Stone Age Diet.

This diet required a person to consume only foods which are considered to be especially safe, and to do this for a period of one to two weeks. For example, one regime was a diet of boiled lamb and pears, while another consisted entirely of vegetables. If the symptoms did not ease after the 7 -14 day trial period, it was concluded that any presenting illness was not allergy-related. If there was an improvement, foods were then carefully re-introduced one at a time on a daily basis and the patient was strictly observed throughout the trial for a return of the symptoms.

Though this test is useful, it has very obvious limitations, the greatest disadvantage being the time it takes. This extended period produces an increasing number of variables which question the practicality and, ultimately, the accuracy of the test. There is also the boredom associated with the dietary restrictions, which can severely test the individual's commitment to it. There are also genuine difficulties associated with fitting this very restricted diet into a busy life for an extended period.

Although this method of allergy-testing has been theoretically considered the "gold standard", it is in most cases a practical impossibility to perform correctly (32). Given these limitations, most people do not see this test as a viable means of identifying food allergies.

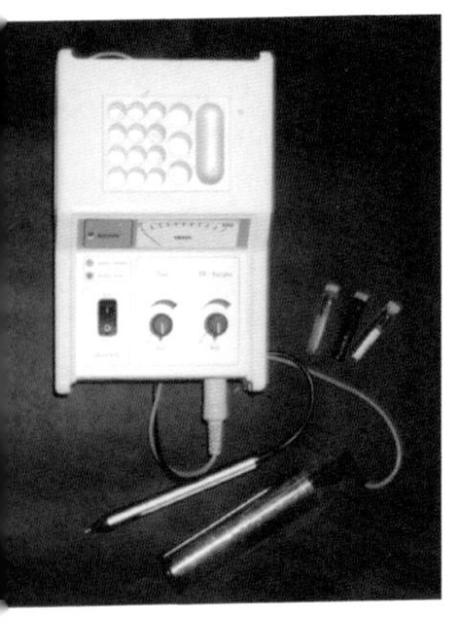

Vega Testing

The Vega machine (known in the US as the Dermatron) is a very sensitive piece of electronic equipment used for measuring comparative resistance. The patient is given an electrode, which acts as an earth, to hold in one hand. A second electrode, designed as a probe, is brought in contact with one of the acupuncture points on the hand. Built into the Vega machine is an ammeter, which crosses the circuit and is then able to get a reading of the meridian electricity which is flowing within the circuit. A special homeopathic allergy test ampoule is then introduced into the circuit and the degree of allergy is interpreted by assessing the degree of distortion recorded on the ammeter.

In my opinion this machine is very difficult to use. Because of the extreme sensitivity of the machine consistent readings are almost impossible to obtain and its record of reproducibility is very poor. Its results also are subject to human interpretation. Finally readings are affected by other factors, including the difficulty of achieving the correct angle or pressure with the probe, the friction it creates, and the intrusion of moisture that results from perspiration. I consider that these factors make the Vega machine unreliable in the diagnosis of food allergies.

Blood Allergy Tests for Slimming

Some organisations use blood allergy tests to assist people to lose weight. Allergies may be associated with problems of overweight, but this is not always the case. The net result of some of these weight loss tests has been to advise people to avoid long lists of food. This is unhelpful because, as mentioned earlier, most people have relatively few primary allergies. The better tests now available are able to pinpoint these primary allergies with accuracy, and it is possible to state that almost 95% of the benefits associated with avoiding allergenic foods are derived from avoiding those classified as a person's primary triggers. And again, it is hard to adhere to a strict regime with so many foods excluded, and people often abandon their prescribed diet after a short period.

In my experience, people who have an overweight problem which is genuinely associated with allergies need only find their two or three primary foods to be able to reap all of the benefits.

Even the Best Tests have Limitations

Even using the best test in the world, and the best designed and best adhered to follow-up programme of food avoidance, not all people presenting with food allergies will be cured. This is because the majority of allergies have a strong emotional component to them. In 75% of cases, the removal of the offending food will stop the symptoms. In the remaining 25% of cases, however, even when the allergic foods are correctly identified and removed from the diet, symptoms will continue, as **excessive stress will keep activating the bowel bacteria to continue to produce toxins** (33). **These toxins are poisonous in their own right and are not dependent on undigested allergic foods to act as a catalyst.** Such situations need more than just allergy testing to resolve the problem. Affected people need to look at every aspect of their health, including any medication which they may be taking, and also to make a serious assessment of the stresses under which they are living.

For details of how to access the IgG test used in my clinic, contact the Clinic Registrar at:

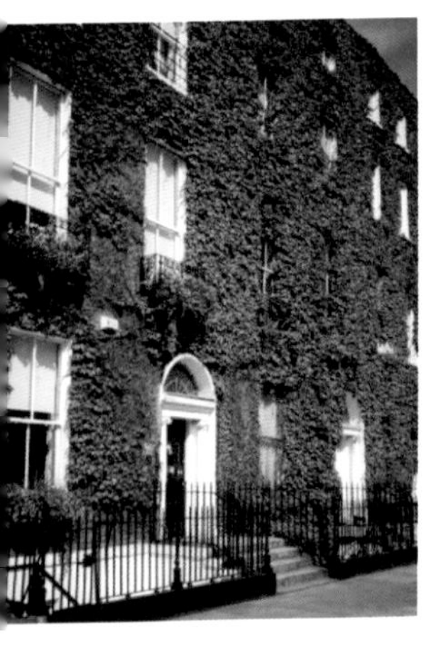

The Fitzwilliam Acupuncture & Allergy Clinic,
68 Fitzwilliam Square North,
Dublin 2,
Ireland
Tel: 00 353 (0)1 661 6082
E-mail: fitzwil@iol.ie

For readers living outsied of Ireland, please refer to the web site listed below for a list of practitioners who wil be able to help you:

Web site: www.martinhealy.com

Chapter Ten

Dairy Products

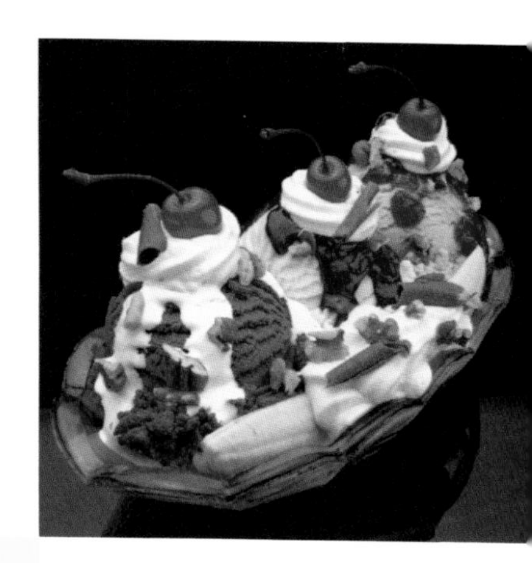

One food group which deserves special attention in the field of allergy investigation is dairy products. Allergy books tend to be either strongly for or strongly against dairy products. My own view is that if you can digest milk, it is perhaps one of the finest and most nutritious foods available. If, on the other hand, you are eating dairy products and your body cannot digest them, they are perhaps one of the most toxic, as even small amounts can trigger serious illness in allergic people.

Why is Cows' Milk the Most Common Allergy Food?

Of all of the foods available to us, cows' milk is perhaps the most complete. It has virtually everything that is required to sustain life. For the first few months of our lives we are able to survive on milk alone. However, because it is such a concentrated food it requires strong digestion to break it down. By contrast, simpler foods such as potato, carrot, rice etc are much easier to digest and rarely cause problems.

Putrefaction and Toxicity

When poorly digested plant matter passes through the digestive tract, it decays with very few undesirable by-products. However, when dairy products which are not properly digested pass through the system, they quickly putrefy within the gut. The putrefaction process produces a number of undesirable toxic by-products, which cause the illnesses associated with dairy allergy.

Lactose Intolerance

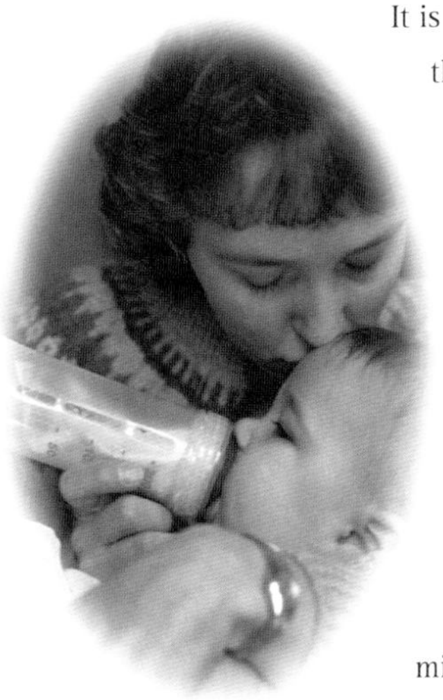

It is generally assumed that lactose – the sugar particles in milk – is the main cause of milk allergy. If these sugar particles are not digested properly, they feed the unfriendly bacteria in the intestines, leading to fermentation, bloating, general discomfort, and possibly diarrhoea or constipation.

In my opinion, however, lactose is not the most problematic part of milk. Around 95% of milk allergy sufferers can drink either goats' milk or skimmed cows' milk as an alternative to whole milk products, and the improvement in their health is often very dramatic. However, both goats' milk and skimmed cows' milk contain lactose. In fact, the lactose count in skimmed milk is even higher than that in ordinary whole milk. This therefore implies that only about 5% of people are allergic to lactose.

In my view the problematic part of milk is the fat content. Undigested dairy fat arriving in the gut interacts with the unfriendly bacteria, creating further toxins which cause dairy allergy reactions.

The 5% of people with milk allergies who have adverse reactions to lactose generally have immediate IgE type reaction – usually swelling of the lip, vomiting or diarrhoea. In most cases, because the reaction follows very soon after eating the offending food, affected people are well aware of the trigger.

Calcium and Osteoporosis

The heated debate often provoked by the suggestion of avoiding dairy products stems from the fear of losing body calcium levels and, as a result, of developing osteoporosis. However, the reality of food allergy is that the body cannot tolerate or process a given kind of food. Having a dairy allergy means that you cannot process the dairy product, which in turn means that you cannot extract the calcium from it. Yet many women who are now suffering with osteoporosis have been depending on and, in many cases, taking extra, dairy products, to increase their calcium levels in the hope of preventing osteoporosis. Because they have been allergic to the dairy products, however, they have not been extracting the calcium. Many women with a confirmed diagnosis of osteoporosis have indeed shown themselves to be allergic to dairy products when tested.

An article in the *British Medical Journal* in January 1986 noted that investigations had revealed that some women who suffer osteoporosis also showed high levels of dairy intolerance. An obvious progression from this study would have been to advise women to reassess their ability to digest dairy products, especially if there was any history of osteoporosis or food allergy within the family. If there was any doubt about the possibility of dairy allergy, they should have been told not to rely on dairy products as their primary source of calcium. This has not so far been done: instead the trend has been to prescribe HRT.

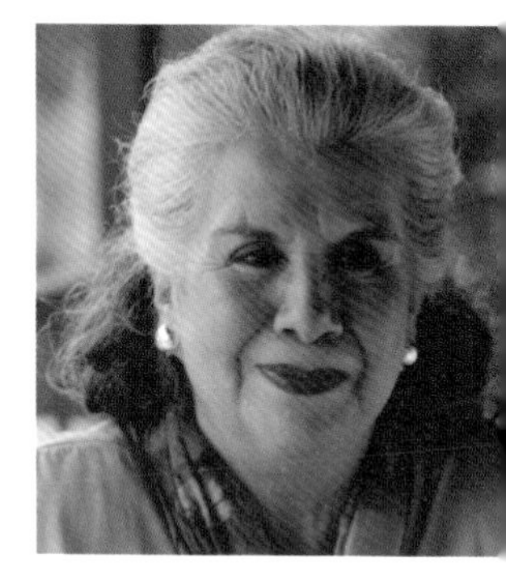

Alternatives to Cows' Milk

For many people switching from full fat to skimmed cows' milk resolves their allergic problem. When a laboratory test report states that you are reacting to cows' milk, it in fact means all dairy products, including:

- yoghurt
- cheese
- milk chocolate
- cream
- ice cream
- butter

Any vegetable spread can be used as a replacement for butter, avoiding, if possible, spreads which use hydrogenated oil. Other options include goats' milk or soya milk products.

It is worth noting, too, that whey, the watery part of the milk that separates from the clot in cheese making, contains much protein and other useful nutrients of milk but none of the fat. Because of this, it rarely causes a problem for dairy-sensitive people.

Goats' Milk

Many people believe that goats' milk is not as nutritious as cows' milk. The reality is that someone with a dairy allergy will obtain more nutrients from drinking water than from cows' milk, to which he or she is allergic. It is worth repeating that if you are allergic to something, not only is it not giving you any nourishment, but it is making you ill.

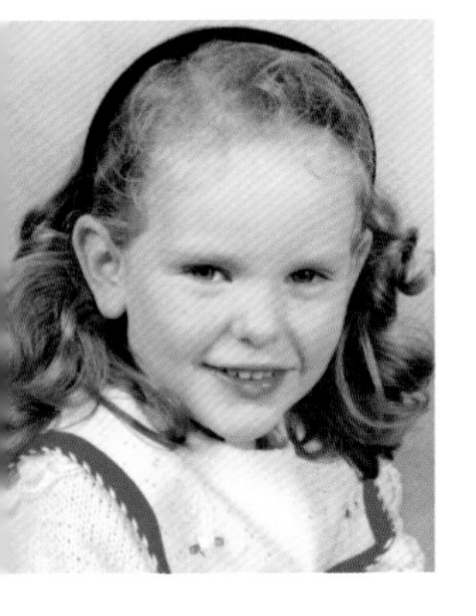

Because goats' milk is stronger in flavour than cows' milk, people sometimes dilute it. This is not good practice in the long run. In introducing goats' milk to children people sometimes water it down a little for the first few days and then gradually build it up to full strength. As a temporary measure this is perfectly fine. I have treated many children who were unable to tolerate cows' milk and as a result were constantly plagued with infections, coughs and colds. By taking them off cows' milk and putting them onto goats' milk, all have thrived. One of my own nieces, Louise, was brought up on goats' milk as a result of recurring ear infections and has now grown into a healthy little girl. She has also now outgrown all her allergies and returned to drinking cows' milk.

Soya Milk

An option open to people allergic to both cows' milk and goats' milk is to use soya milk. In this case it is perhaps better to use soya milk which is supplemented with calcium, as soya is fairly heavily processed and may have lost some of its natural calcium content. Use a product which does not have sugar added to the milk as this leads to problems of tooth decay. Another possibility is rice milk.

Yoghurt

Yoghurt is increasingly being recognised for its therapeutic value. It is the friendly bacteria it contains which gives yoghurt its therapeutic edge. Many products are now promoted as "Bio" yoghurt; this simply means that yoghurt cultures have been added at some stage in the manufacturing process. However, if the yoghurt is heat-treated (pasteurised) after the cultures have been added, the bacteria will be killed. It is best to buy yoghurt which is guaranteed to be "live". This places responsibility on the manufacturer to ensure that the cultures are indeed live when you purchase the yoghurt.

Recommended Therapeutic Cultures

Of the cultures available to us bifidobacteria are the most useful. Other yoghurt cultures include:

- Lactobacillus acidophilus;
- Bifidobacterium longum;
- Lactobacillus Bulgaricus;
- Streptococcus thermophilus.

To get the best from yoghurt you should pay close attention to where it comes from and how it is made. Some points to consider:

- All yoghurt cultures require great attention to detail in every aspect of manufacture, transportation and shelf storage. Because they are so fragile, their life span is very short outside their natural environment of the intestines. Only the very best quality products made by the very best manufacturers, and "guaranteed live", are of any real value. Cultures sold over the counter can also be past their best and, as a consequence, of little benefit.
- To check if your particular brand of yoghurt really is live, take a few tablespoons of the yoghurt and mix it with a cup of regular milk which has been heated but not boiled. Leave this overnight in a warm place, such as a hot-press. By morning, if the original really was live, it will have thickened.

- These cultures only work well when stress, antibiotics, steroids, allergic foods and other triggers have been attended to. Otherwise, within a very short space of time, the unfriendly bacteria in the intestines will be reactivated and everything will revert back to where it started.

- If you want to be sure of fresh, live yoghurt, make your own with skimmed milk and a special culture mix. Rather than buy fruit-flavoured yoghurt, in which the fruit is often processed with chemicals, buy natural live yoghurt and add real fresh fruit at the time of eating.

- Remember that even the best quality live yoghurt is of no benefit to you if you have a serious dairy allergy. In fact it will make you more ill.

Importance of Calcium Supplementation

The calcium content of fruit and vegetables, including the humble potato, is very high. Most important of all is the fact that these foods are "simple" – that is, easily processed by the digestive system. This means that the calcium is easily extracted by the body and absorbed into the system. Fruits and vegetables high in calcium include rhubarb, figs, raspberries, green leafy vegetables, beans and legumes, as well as sesame seeds and nuts.

Because people who suffer with food allergies are on restricted diets, however, it is often essential to assist them with appropriate supplements. Because calcium is such a vital constituent of bones and teeth, and because dairy products, when we are not allergic to them, are among the best available sources of calcium, I recommend that all people who have a confirmed allergy to dairy products take such a calcium supplement daily.

Vitamins and minerals are available to us in two forms, inorganic (chemical) and organic (food state). Nature's process is to convert the inorganic vitamins and minerals into organic form through the growing of plants in the soil. The plant is then eaten by humans and the organic vitamins and minerals are readily available. The majority of supplements sold to the public are inorganic and as a result, are less appropriate for the human tissues. Look for "Food State" supplements manufactured by a company called "Nature's Own".

Such supplements are as close to food sources as possible: for example, Vitamin C supplements are complexed in fruit pulp made from oranges, and betacarotene is complexed in carrot concentrate. Food state calcium supplements are also available. Studies have shown that the body absorbs supplements manufactured in this way significantly more readily.

Note: Take calcium supplements with food, and never on an empty stomach.

A Word of Caution to Vegetarians

People who do not eat meat often rely on dairy products for their protein and other essential nutrients, so problems arise when vegetarians become allergic to dairy products. It is my opinion that the vegetarian approach in such cases is not to be recommended. The diet becomes too restricted and the potential of developing nutritional deficiencies becomes a real possibility.

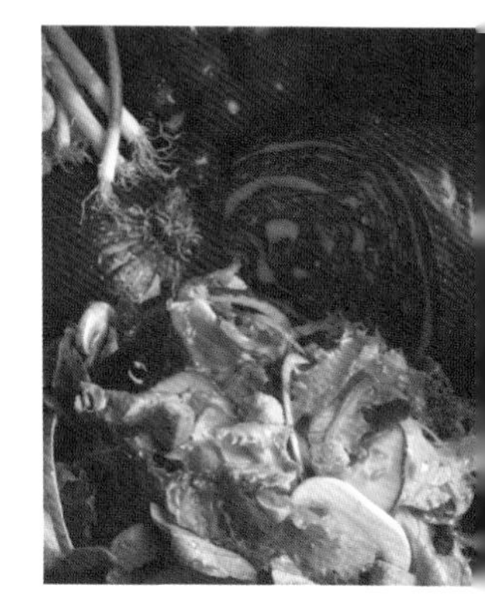

Chapter Eleven

17 Food Profiles

17 key foods listed with an outline of their specific nutritional benefits as well as their associated allergy risks

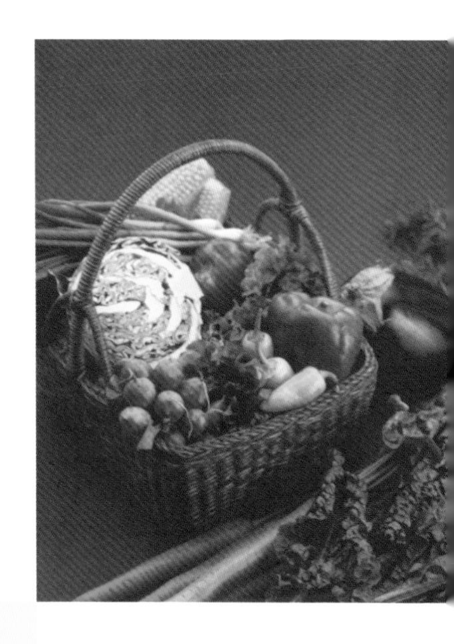

Of all the foods that are available to us only a small group is particularly associated with allergies. The foods considered in this chapter deserve special comment. The reader should nevertheless keep in mind that all comments about the foods in this section relate to slow-reaction food allergies. People who have sensitivities to these delayed-response foods, or aspects of them, can in many instances tolerate them in moderation. This chapter tells you about which aspects of these foods generally cause the reaction and suggests alternatives.

None of this applies to people suffering with classical (IgE related) allergies, since even a very small amount can bring on potentially life-threatening reactions. **If you have classical (IgE) allergy reactions you should never eat the food in any form.**

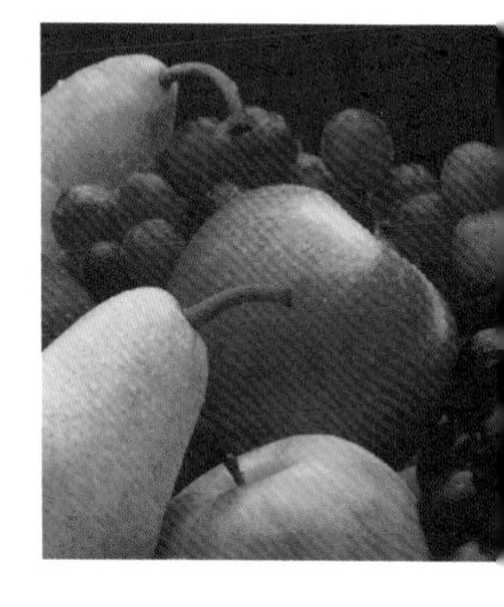

Nutrients in Fruit and Vegetables

Before looking at these foods selected for their association with slow-response food allergies, it is worth referring to an article which appeared in *Newsweek* (April 25, 1994) discussing the significance of some newly discovered food nutrients called phytochemicals.

Unavailable to us at present except inside natural foods, these compounds are proving to be among the most important nutrients yet discovered in our food. Every slice of every fruit and vegetable contains thousands of different phytochemical compounds which provide fruits and vegetables with specific protection. This protection is in turn passed onto those who eat them.

In the United States, the National Cancer Institute is currently proposing a multimillion-dollar project to isolate phytochemicals. Private companies are said to be eyeing them as a health blockbuster. Among their most interesting properties is the apparent ability to block the chain of events which ultimately lead to cancer. A senior health adviser in the U.S. Public Health Service is quoted as saying that "these natural products can take tumours and diffuse them. They can turn off the proliferation process of cancer". (*Newsweek*, April 25, 1994)

Recently, researchers identified the cancer-preventing potential of one of these phytochemicals, named sulforaphane, which is found in broccoli, cauliflower, brussels sprouts, turnips and kale. Researchers at John Hopkins Medical Institution have found that it offers powerful protection against cancer in animals. Laboratory experiments on human cells showed that sulforaphane boosted the synthesis of cancer-destroying enzymes. Especial good news is that neither microwaving nor cooking destroys sulforaphane. Researchers have found that within hours of the broccoli arriving in the stomach, it begins a process of literally carting the carcinogen out of the cell.

Cancer is a multi-step process. Cells go through many changes before they arrive at the malignancy stage. According to epidemiologist Dr. John Potter of the University of Minnesota, "at almost every one of the steps along the pathway leading to cancer there are one or more compounds in vegetables or fruit that will slow up or reverse the process".

Research suggests that juices and extracts are not as beneficial as the whole fruit or vegetable in terms of phytochemical protection. The more you eat, and the more variety of fruit and vegetables you are able to include in what you eat, the better.

The phytochemicals which have been discovered so far are only the tip of the iceberg, but their discovery reconfirms the instinct that suggests that the natural, whole food is best. This is why I am leading you back to the dining table in your quest to track the cause of your illness. Equally, it is here that you may well find the cure for your illness. Allergy testing can specify which food is to be avoided, after which you can safely eat a cross-section of foods which will supply your body with the range of nutrients it needs. In this way you can assist your body in its journey back to good health.

Each of the foods considered in this chapter can be life-enhancing when you can digest it and potentially poisonous when you cannot. It is important to remember that if you cannot digest something properly – even the most natural and nutritious food – actually it will be doing you harm.

Wheat

Much of what you have heard from consultants and read in health magazines goes out the window for many people who have irritable bowel syndrome (IBS). The advice coming from both of these sources is to eat lots of roughage in the form of wheat bran, high-fibre breakfast cereals and wholemeal bread to assist the condition. While this is the correct advice for some people, a significant proportion of IBS sufferers are actually allergic to wheat. For the person suffering from wheat sensitivity, it has been my experience that it is the bran – the coarse, roughage component – that provokes the reaction.

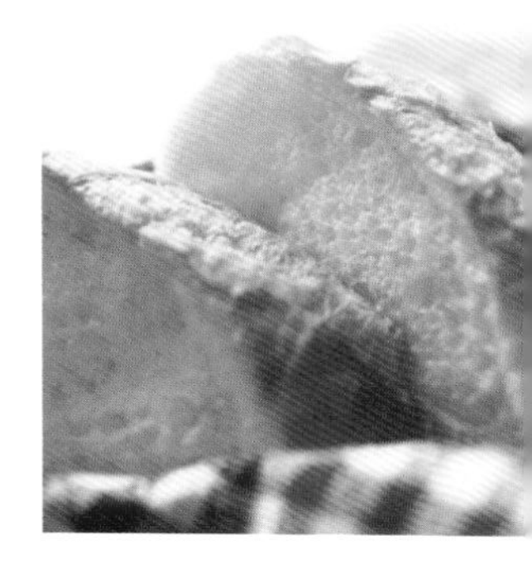

Bread

Wheat-sensitive people do not necessarily have to stop eating bread altogether, however. Experience has taught me that it is the wholemeal, high-fibre breads and, the other extreme, the very fresh and "doughy" breads, which cause the reaction. A moderate intake of a light in-between bread may be alright for you. Light "slimming" breads are a possibility, but have the disadvantage of being made with processed wheat, which has lost much of its nutritional value. Another alternative would be to eat a rye bread. Rye makes a very heavy flour and as a result 100% rye bread can be unpalatable. Most bakers use a half rye, half wheat mixture in their rye bread. Experiment a little with these varieties of bread to find your own tolerance level.

Alternative Carbohydrates

Wheat-sensitive people should incorporate another cereal into their diet to compensate for the reduction in bread consumption. They should increase the intake of oat, rice or corn breakfast cereals; potatoes; rice; and rice or corn pasta. Other cereals, vegetables and fruit should be eaten to ensure adequate roughage in the diet. Ordinary pasta, made with "doughy" wheat, should be avoided, and commercial breakfast cereals checked for wheat content. Nuts, oat biscuits, popcorn, potato and other crisps and the like, could be eaten as substitutes for biscuits and cakes which contain wheat flour.

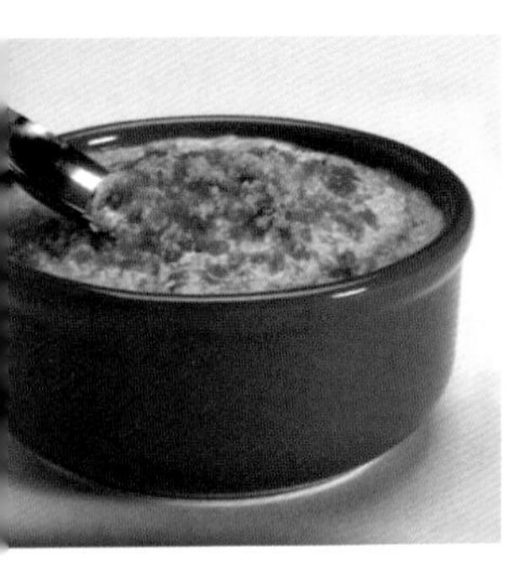

Oats

Oats are the least refined of all available breakfast cereals; they are filling but also easy to digest. They contain fibre, can lower cholesterol, and help to stabilise blood glucose levels. They are traditionally associated with supporting the nervous system.

Rice

Rice is one of the least allergenic foods. Brown rice is particularly nutritious and high in fibre but it should perhaps be avoided in favour of white rice by people who have IBS. Rice gives a gentler rise in blood sugar than potatoes or bread.

Yeast

Yeast is a type of vegetable micro-organism which produces fermentation. It is used in baking bread and in the production of alcohol.

Allergies to yeast are at the very core of the mechanism which lies behind many food sensitivities. Some people have an excess of particular yeasts in their intestine, and the consumption of extra yeast –

or foods which directly feed and encourage these intestinal yeasts – causes overload in the system, and this triggers allergic reactions.

If your laboratory test results return with a strong positive reaction to yeast you must avoid foods:

- With a strong yeast content – notably alcoholic drinks and bread;
- Which directly feed the yeast – notably sugar.

Alcoholic drinks with a strong yeast content include fermented drinks such as beer, lager, stout and wine. These need to be substituted by distilled alcoholic drinks, such as whiskey, brandy, gin and vodka.

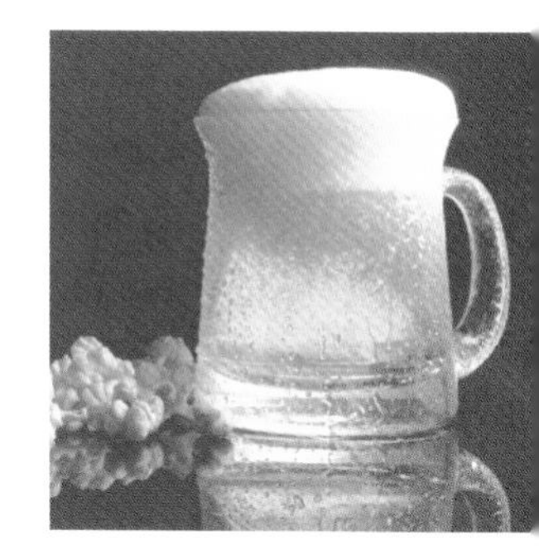

Yeast is used to provide the "lift" for bread dough. However, many commercial breads contain minimum yeast as it is now the practice to pump air under pressure through the dough mixture to achieve lift. The small amount of yeast in most kinds of bread is mostly killed off during the baking process; so people with yeast allergies can often eat small amounts of light commercial breads. Each person has to find his or her own tolerance level.

Many people who react adversely to yeast eat heavy, wholemeal, yeast-free bread, for example soda and sour-dough bread, as an alternative. This, however, is not helpful, as the roughage in these kinds of bread feeds and encourages intestinal yeast. Note also that dairy fat directly encourages the growth of intestinal yeast. People who are allergic to yeast should also avoid dairy fat.

Increase your fruit and vegetable intake to compensate for the roughage lost by reducing wholemeal varieties of bread.

Soya

Soya is the traditional substitute for people who have slow-response allergies to dairy products. For vegetarians it is often the primary substitute for meat. However, in recent years I have observed that soya is increasingly causing allergy reactions. Soya is one of the foods which have been most subjected to genetic engineering. Whether the increasing number of confirmed allergy reactions to soya is the result of genetic engineering or merely of more sensitive testing procedures, is difficult to say.

The genetic engineering of plants consists in transferring genes from one plant to another, or from an animal to a plant and vice versa. The gene in question endows the host with specific characteristics. One example of this is the splicing of a gene from a fish into a tomato to give the tomato a longer shelf-life. This, however, is potentially disastrous for anyone with an allergy to fish. The person in question could be made severely ill by eating these genetically-modified tomatoes but be quite unable to account for this reaction. In effect, the practice of genetic engineering is fraught with danger for the allergy sufferer.

Soya beans, as flour or starch, feature as ingredients in a wide variety of foods, from bread and baked goods to salad dressings and sauces. Also commonly used are oil and other soya derivatives. People with strong allergies to soya need to be very vigilant.

Traditionally soya has been relied upon as a good source of calcium for those unable to tolerate dairy products. However, because of genetic engineering and processing, it is difficult to know if it is still as reliable a source. Many manufacturers now supplement their soya milk products with extra calcium. Another safeguard is to use organically produced soya products.

Tofu

This versatile food product looks like a block of cheese. It is made with soya set by calcium chloride and is the richest non-dairy source of calcium.

Beef

People with strong allergies to dairy products need to exercise caution with beef. The fat content of the dairy produce, which causes the reaction, is also to be found within the meat.

The best alternatives are fish, chicken, turkey and the leanest cuts of lamb. Most of the fat of the chicken or turkey is in the skin so avoid eating this also.

Eggs

Eggs are a high-protein food which putrefies in the intestines if it is not properly digested. Few people need to be reminded of the unbearable smell of an egg which has gone off. But this is exactly what happens when you eat eggs if you are allergic to them. Next to dairy products I regard eggs as the second most toxic food to the human body when a person is allergic to it.

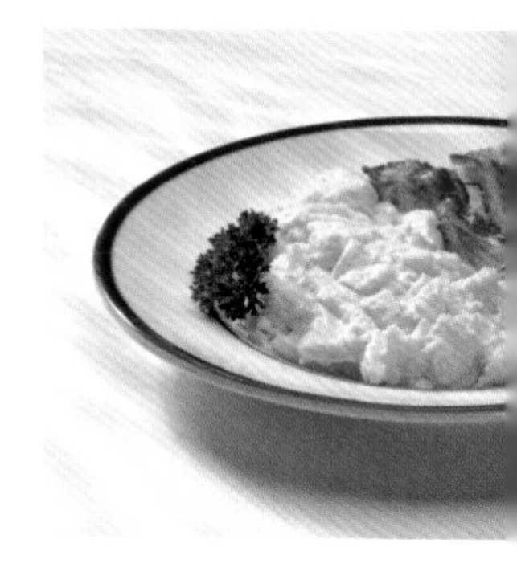

Good allergy tests are able to distinguish between sensitivity reactions to egg white and egg yolk. Evidence indicates that it is the egg white which is more likely to be allergenic. People with this allergy need therefore also to avoid such foods as meringues, souffles and cake icing, which contains egg white.

For those allergic to egg yolk, this is an ingredient in mayonnaise, salad cream and pasta.

Cakes and Biscuits

While people who have classical allergy reactions to eggs must never eat them in any form, commercial egg substitute, which many manufacturers use in cakes and biscuits, does not have the same potential to trigger reactions in people with delayed response allergy to eggs. For many people with this kind of allergy reaction to eggs, a low to moderate intake of commercially-produced cakes and biscuits should not be a problem. Home-made cakes containing two or more whole eggs, should be avoided, however.

Cholesterol

Because of the association between egg and high cholesterol levels it is perhaps wise even for those without allergies or sensitivities to egg, to restrict them to a maximum of three per week.

Cautionary Note

Many vaccines are grown on an egg culture and may cause reactions. If you know that you have any kind of allergic reaction to eggs, you must always tell your doctor, especially before having a vaccination.

Oily Fish

Eating more oily fish, such as salmon, mackerel, herring, trout and sardines, is to be recommended for a variety of reasons. Oils in these fish contain special fats known as essential fatty acids (EFA) which are linked to a myriad of health benefits.

EFAs are found in polyunsaturated fats, which the human body cannot produce on its own, so it is important to eat some of them. Unlike saturated and trans fats, which are associated with heart and circulatory disease, polyunsaturated fats are beneficial to health.

The Nurses' Health Study

A well-respected and well-known study by a professional nursing organisation which followed over 80,000 women for a period of fourteen years, found that for each increase of five per cent of saturated fat, there was an associated seventeen per cent increase in the risk of coronary artery disease. The survey also showed that the replacement of saturated, hydrogenated fats with non-hydrogenated, polyunsaturated fats was more effective in preventing coronary artery disease than simply reducing the overall saturated fat intake.

Shellfish

Shellfish are almost as nutritious as oily fish – high in EFAs and iodine – but rate very high in their potential to trigger allergies, especially the fast acting, violent IgE type. Because shellfish usually trigger only the (IgE) response, the IgG test may give the "all clear" when in fact you may have a major problem with shellfish.

Note: What applies to shellfish applies to peanuts. Always seek the advice of a competent practitioner if you are in any doubt.

Beans and Lentils

Dried beans and lentils (pulses) are nutritious and important in any diet. They are rich in iron and fibre; their high potassium content helps regulate blood pressure; and they can also reduce blood cholesterol levels substantially.

The allergenic potential of beans and lentils is relatively low. However, their tendency to produce wind can be a problem for some. Adequate soaking overnight and the addition of herbs and spices such as fennel seeds and dill help reduce this flatulent effect.

Potato

Potatoes are a highly recommended food as they rarely trigger slow-response food allergies. They are highly nutritious, being rich in calcium and potassium and a good source of fibre. Eat them with their jackets on as the majority of the nutrients are situated just underneath the skin, and use a non-hydrogenated vegetable spread instead of butter.

Sweet potato contains more nutrients than the unrelated ordinary potato. As with the ordinary potato, by far the majority of the nutrients are just under the skin. So do not peel them before cooking; scrub them thoroughly instead.

Onion

The many health benefits attributed to the onion – lowering blood pressure and cholesterol levels, helping with coughs and colds – are associated with the volatile enzymes and strong smells which are released when they are freshly chopped. It is therefore best to use only fresh onions when cooking. Commercially prepared onion products have lost much of this nutritional vitality and therapeutic potential.

Many people with onion sensitivity say that they only react to raw onions and that well-cooked onions do not cause them a problem. It appears that cooking alters the element within the onion which causes the reaction.

Garlic

Garlic shares with the onion a very strong pungent nature. Its therapeutic potential is similar to that of the onion in that it is useful for treating infections, especially of the chest, blood and general circulation. It has double the therapeutic potential of the onion and this makes it a very useful therapeutic agent.

Many people with chest infections who dislike the taste of garlic make dramatic improvements on high doses of odourless garlic pearls.

Note: In all cases of infection, and as an added safeguard, it is best to always seek the advice of a competent practitioner.

Citrus Fruit

All citrus fruits provide valuable quantities of vitamin C. The fact that they are generally eaten uncooked ensures that none of the vitamin is lost. Drinking commercial orange or grapefruit juices is not as nutritious as eating the whole, fresh fruit.

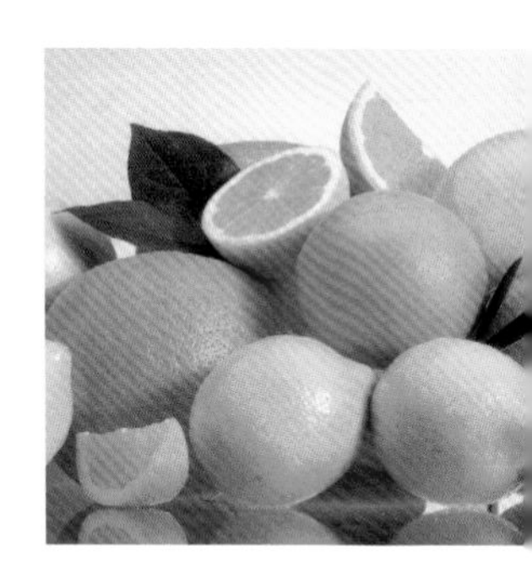

If you are allergic to citrus you can still eat other ripe fruits. Most fruits are slightly acidic when they are not ripe. However, as the fruit ripens, levels of the natural fruit sugars (fructose) overtake those of the acids and quickly neutralise them.

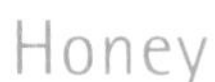

Honey

Honey is for us one of the great gifts of nature, as it gathers together the essences of many different flowers and plants. Of particular interest is honey's ability to kill bacteria. In this respect it is particularly useful in assisting with a wide range of conditions, including coughs and colds, burns, respiratory and sinus infections.

Honey is particularly rich in vitamin C; several B vitamins; amino acids; and citric acid, potassium, calcium, iron, copper, manganese, phosphorus and magnesium. All of these boost the immune system, enabling it to fight infection. In addition it also contains inhibitors which render bacteria harmless. Tests have shown, in particular, that honey has the potential to kill helicobacter pylori, the bacterium associated with stomach ulcers.

Many people who suffer with hayfever or pollen-induced asthma find relief by using honeycomb or cold-pressed honey. The pollen in unfiltered honey seems to have a desensitizing effect on sufferers. To build up resistance you need to use honey all through the pollen season, starting one month before the season begins.

Most honey is heat-treated to help to filter it, delay solidification and speed jar-filling. However, heating reduces some of the antibiotic properties of honey. Even the best honey will suffer in quality when used in cooking or baking or when stored in the refrigerator.

It is not advisable to to give honey to infants under one year old as allergic reactions, though rare, are not unknown. It should not be overlooked also that honey causes tooth decay almost as quickly as sugar.

Tea and Coffee

Tea and coffee have in recent times been blamed for many common ailments. The stimulant aspect of the caffeine content of both causes most of the problem, so many manufacturers are now producing decaffeinated teas and coffees. However, decaffeinating tea and coffee is a serious chemical process, which can in itself be a problem. It has been my experience that if a person shows a positive allergic reaction to tea or coffee, changing to decaffeinated does not help.

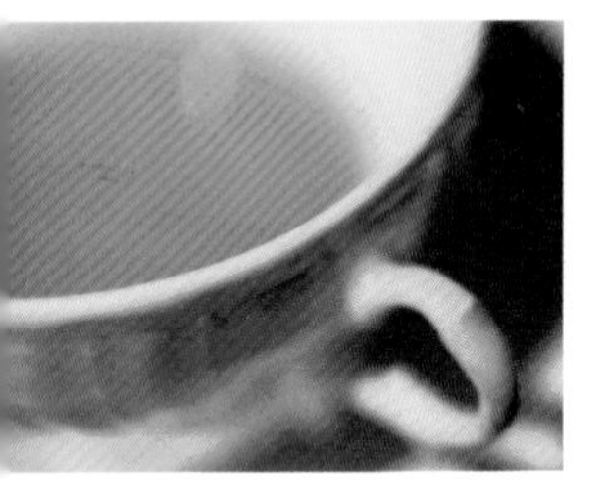

The stimulant potential of coffee is very strong and it is wise for everyone to keep consumption to a minimum – a maximum of three cups per day for people who are not allergic to it. Caffeine has an unsettling effect on the nervous system. Mild instant coffees are less harmful than percolated coffee, especially when diluted with milk.

Tea is also a mild stimulant. It rarely shows positive on the allergy test and is fine for most people. However, it is best not to drink it very strong. Tea also contains anti-oxidants which help the immune system to fight poisons and assist the breakdown of fats after a meal.

Herbal teas are another "healthy" option, especially camomile, as it has a gentle relaxing effect upon the system.

Cola Nut

The cola (kola) nut is another caffeine-rich stimulant and one of the main ingredients in cola drinks. It is its caffeine content that poses a problem for the allergy sufferer. It is also used therapeutically in cough syrups as a means of opening the bronchial tubes.

In addition to those who show a positive allergic reaction to the cola nut, pregnant women; people suffering from insomnia, chronic high blood pressure, high cholesterol, heart disease; and those who have a history of stroke should avoid cola and other caffeine-rich food and drinks.

Chapter Twelve

Five Element Acupuncture

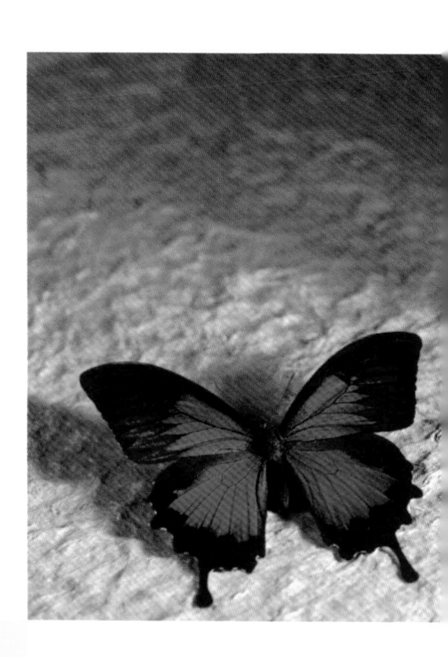

A small percentage of people, even after they have found and avoided their allergenic foods, will not improve significantly. Of those who do improve, some will be interested in investigating a treatment system which may assist them further with their own particular allergy tendencies and also help to build up resistance against any future allergies. It is my belief that Five Element Acupuncture is ideally suited to assist both sets of people to return to full health. This is because it is focused on assisting people to manage better the stress in their lives. There are many different styles of acupuncture, each with its own emphasis. Five Element Acupuncture is in my view the most effective style for treating allergy-related problems. It is also very fast acting, achieving noticeable results within three to four treatments in most cases.

Some Notes on the History of Acupuncture

Acupuncture has been practised in China for at least 2,000 years. The practice spread to other countries in the East and, as it did, individual interpretations and styles of application began to emerge.

With the encouragement of the Communist authorities after 1948, a new development in traditional Chinese medicine was instituted. It became known as Traditional Chinese Medicine (TCM). This modern development of acupuncture has been strongly influenced by Western medical thinking. Like Western medicine, TCM is more focused on the external causative factors of disease. In particular it emphasises the effect of the climatic factors of dampness, wind and cold. TCM tends to focus more upon patterns of disharmony within the physical body, and diagnosis is made by observing how aspects of this disharmony manifest as disease. It is now practised in much of China and the rest of the world, and while it draws on ancient traditions it is largely a creation of the second half of the twentieth century (34).

Five Element Acupuncture is, by contrast, more focused on the emotional causative factors of disease. The *Nei Jing*, a book written 2,000 years ago and treated as almost the bible of traditional oriental medicine, emphasises this association. Written in the form of a series of dialogues between the Yellow Emperor and his court physician,Qi Bo, the *Nei Jing* emphasises the connection between disease and the stresses and worries of people. For example, the Yellow Emperor asks of his physician:

> *"In ancient times disease was cured by prayer alone. . . but nowadays physicians treat disease with herbs . . . and acupuncture . . . and the disease is sometimes cured and sometimes not cured. Why? Qi Bo answered: The ancient people lived . . . with neither internal burden of wishes and envies nor external burden of chasing after fame and profit, it was a life of tranquillity which made them immune from the deep intrusion of vicious energies. . . Nowadays. . . they worry a great deal, they work too hard, they fail to follow the climates. . . they have lowered their moral standards, with the results that they are under the attack of vicious energies frequently . . . and when the patient's spirits are not positive, and when their will and sentiments are not stable, the disease cannot recover."*

The *Nei Jing* contains many examples which testify to the careful attention these ancient practitioners gave to the emotional life of their patients.

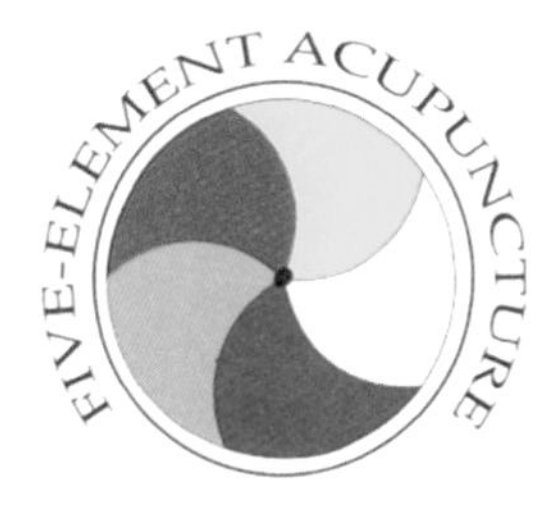

Five Element Acupuncture

One man who did more than any to bring this particular style to the West is Professor J.R. Worsley (see Appendix 1).

Basic Principles of Acupuncture

Traditionally, acupuncture has been explained in terms of an energy system. It was proposed that energy circulates within the body via a series of channels called meridians, controlling the functioning of all organs and body systems. Disease is said to appear as a result of a blockage or other disturbance of these channels. Western medicine would perhaps see these channels as being in some way connected to, or associated with, the nervous system.

Acupuncture is often explained in terms of c'hi, yin and yang and the five elements, reflecting the language and the belief systems of its origins. My own view is that the literal interpretation of this language, and its use in present-day acupuncture practice, creates confusion and that we would do better to translate it into the language of our times.

The Acupuncture–Immune System Connection

The most straightforward translation I can offer for the idea of an energy system within the body is that it is closely associated with the autonomic nervous system. This aspect of the nervous system is known to exercise a strong influence over the immune system. Acupuncture practitioners say that they are able to influence the immune system as a result of manipulating these autonomic-system energy lines.

Until the beginning of the twentieth century a somewhat similar view was to be found in Western medicine in that it was assumed that electrical impulses from the nervous system were responsible for all physiological functioning. Then a substance in the body which stimulates the pancreas to produce digestive enzymes was discovered. This new substance was classified as a hormone, and was the first of many to be found.

Hormones are chemical messengers which trigger a specific response in organs and systems of the body. Their effect on a particular organ or body system is very much like a car key fitting into the ignition and starting the engine.

Recently, Dr. Candice Pert, who has worked for many years as a research scientist at the US National Institute of Health, the country's leading health research establishment, discovered a new group of hormones. Her book *Molecules of Emotion* (35) describes how the emotional part of the brain is a storehouse for many of these hormones. The brain sends out these hormones to communicate with the organs and body systems. In addition to autonomic nerve reflexes, these hormone messengers appear to be the primary driving force behind the entire body.

It is my belief that the system that the ancient Chinese practitioners called energy channels is the common link between these autonomic nerve reflexes and the hormonal messenger system. I base this belief on the understanding that the organs and systems that are directly affected by these hormones and nerve reflexes are the same organs and systems that are affected by acupuncture. **Using acupuncture we are, I believe, able to adjust and rebalance the combined effects of these two systems.**

In Pert's work, science is for the first time describing the interconnection between body and mind, and explaining how emotionally triggered hormones and the autonomic nervous system affect the workings of the body. This contrasts with the predominant model of Western medicine which has focused on the development of specialist knowledge of each body system, rather than looking at how the whole system fits together as a whole and works as one integrated unit. A case can be made, however, to say that focusing on and treating one specific body system in isolation from the whole organism is misleading and can lead to inaccurate diagnosis and inappropriate treatments.

A prime example of this occurs when a person is adversely affected by stress and anxiety caused by emotional problems. This leads to the release of high levels of the hormone adrenaline, triggering a rapid heart beat and high blood pressure. Such patients are sent to the cardiologist, whose sole focus is on the condition of the heart and blood vessels. By means of powerful medication the cardiologist is able to bring blood pressure and heart rate under control, but the patient's anxiety remains, and the real cause of the disease is missed.

I believe that many of the conditions that people endure are not diseases *per se* but, like the example above, are, rather, the end result of a whole series of problems which have been troubling the person concerned. A chain of events is set in motion which ultimately manifests in the physical body as illness or disease. This is why in many conditions medication only contains the problem and does not cure it. When the person stops taking the medication, the condition returns. This is perhaps a frightening indictment of much of what Western medicine is about, but it is a reality to which we should face up.

Consulting an Acupuncture Practitioner

There are twelve pathways which make up the complete energy circuit of the body. Energy surges from one pathway into the next through a series of gates known as "entry–exit" points, in the same way that gates along a canal control the flow of water. People who have allergies tend to develop major blocks around these gates. Much of the initial work involves using needles at these specific entry-exit points to clear the blockage. This allows the vital energy to cascade onwards towards arid and depleted areas of the body. Any treatment that does not first clear these blocks will normally not benefit the patient.

Perhaps the greatest breakthrough associated with ancient acupuncture was the discovery of a method of reading how the overall circuit was flowing. The method used is referred to as pulse diagnosis. Twelve different pulse phenomena are discernible, six on each wrist, palpated on the radial artery. Each position reflects the state of charge within each of the twelve main energy pathways, enabling practitioners to get an overall view of the state of charge. Pulse diagnosis takes many years to learn and requires continuous practice. It is the vital component of this style of treatment because the selection of points and all subsequent treatment plans are based on these readings.

Another very important aspect of the Five Element diagnostic approach is the identifying of which emotion is most disturbed and then the treating of the corresponding meridian pathway to calm that troubled emotion. How this is done is beyond the scope of this book. Interested readers should refer to the bibliography.

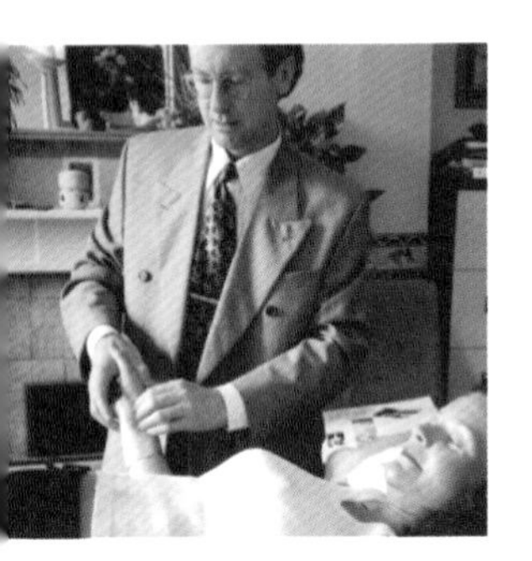

The Acupuncture Points

As described above, acupuncture points are like canal gates in that they control the flow of nerve energy and hormone messengers around the body. The points are graded according to the amount of control they can exert over this flow. As well as "entry-exit" points there are "command points". These are situated between elbow and hand and between knee and foot, and are vitally important in the treatment of allergy-related problems. They are called command points because they have the most control over the entire energy pathway system. When a person is being treated for allergies, these are the areas of the body that are most frequently worked upon.

The technique used by the practitioner determines whether the meridian flow needs to be increased or decreased. Generally speaking, leaving the needle in place for a set period of time tends to sedate or slow the flow, and inserting the needle to stimulate the point and immediately removing it tends to tonify or increase the flow.

The points run very close to the skin surface and as a result very shallow needle penetration is all that is required. All acupuncture needles are used only once and are then thrown away. They are made of high quality stainless steel and in many cases are as fine as the hair on one's head. Because they are so fine, considerable skill is required to insert them. This also means that the whole procedure is practically painless. All that is felt is a particular mild numbness or tingling sensation.

Length of Treatment

Practitioners of Five Element Acupuncture usually allocate between forty-five minutes to one hour for each treatment session.

If the acupuncture treatment is going to work the patient should feel a definite improvement within three to four treatments. Obviously, the more chronic the condition, the more difficult it is to cure. However, in general, if there is no improvement by perhaps the fourth visit, the person should discontinue treatment.

With patients who are responding, the normal procedure is to begin to space out the treatments once a sustained improvement has been established. Each practitioner has his or her own way of working but normally treatment extends from fortnightly visits to monthly and then three monthly visits. Thereafter, any future treatments depend upon how the patient is progressing and how well overall improvement is maintained.

Some medical insurance companies now offer cover for acupuncture and certain other forms of complementary medicine. Enquire about this from your medical insurer.

Obstacles to Progress of Treatment

Severe food allergies are in my view one of the most powerful blocks to the progress of acupuncture treatment and yet they have gone almost totally unrecognized. Why should this be so?

Acupuncture aims to restore and rebalance the energy circuit of the body by stimulating specific aspects of the meridian pathways.

However, if the body is to respond to the energetic stimulation of acupuncture it must firstly be able to react. If its reactive capability is depressed, for whatever reason, the ability to make significant improvements is severely compromised. It is as if the source of that healing power within the body cannot be contacted.

Apart from very severe or terminal illness, which literally overwhelms the system, the three main causes of poor reactive capability are:

- Suppressive drug therapy (especially steroids).
- Very severe stress over a prolonged period of time.
- Food allergies.

The suppressive effects of steroids are well documented and understood within orthodox and complementary medicine alike. They are often used in allergy-related conditions to block the associated inflammatory reaction. This process, however, is in fact a part of the defence response of the immune system. Steroids appear to have the effect of suppressing the immune system. From the point of view of acupuncture treatment, in which effort is principally directed towards supporting and stimulating the body's immune system, suppressive therapies are a contradiction in terms, in most cases rendering treatment null and void.

It has been my experience that strong allergies have a similarly suppressive effect on the immune system. Many patients with strong allergies fail to respond to acupuncture treatment.

I first observed this in the mid-1980s when I was introduced to the curative potential of allergy testing. I had a group of patients at that time who were not making progress with acupuncture treatments. I noticed that this group consisted primarily of people who suffered from conditions believed (but not proven) to have a strong allergy component. I decided to have these people tested and treated for allergies and observed how they progressed.

Within one to three weeks of being on an allergy diet, the majority began to improve. I then restarted the patients' acupuncture treatments and observed their progress.

One thing which all these patients shared during their acupuncture treatment prior to the allergy testing and subsequent modified diets was a reduced ability to feel the sensations patients normally feel from the acupuncture needles. In normal cases when the acupuncture needle makes contact with the acupuncture point, it produces a sensation which patients describe as a dulling, numbing or mildly tingling sensation. Practitioners often refer to this sensation as "dai chi", which translates as "the particular sensation experienced when the energy arrives at the needle". It has to be experienced to be fully understood. In my experience unless the practitioner is able to evoke this sensation in the patient, it is unlikely that the acupuncture will be of benefit.

When I first started to treat this group of patients with acupuncture, I noticed it was very difficult for me to sense that I had made contact with their acupuncture points: these people experienced very little dai chi. However, once the allergic foods had been removed from their diet, they began to experience the needle sensation clearly and strongly; they also began to show significantly more improvement. It became clear to me that allergic foods have a suppressive effect upon the immune system.

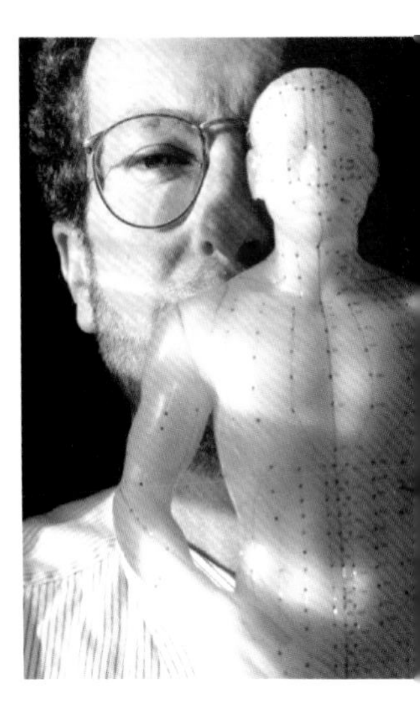

Photos courtesy of Frank Miller, The Irish Times

Energetic Recordings

Advances in medical technology now allow us to record much of the electrical activity within the body. For example, an EEG (electroencephalogram) records the electrical activity of the brain. The meridian circuit is very similar to the EEG circuit in that it also transmits a minute electrical current. This charge can be recorded on an instrument known as the Segmental Electrogram, which, like the EEG machine, gives a print-out of its recordings.

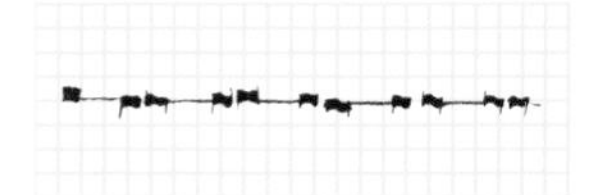

Diagram 1

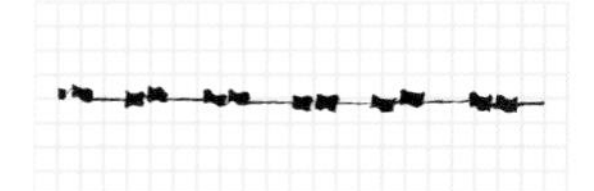

Diagram 2

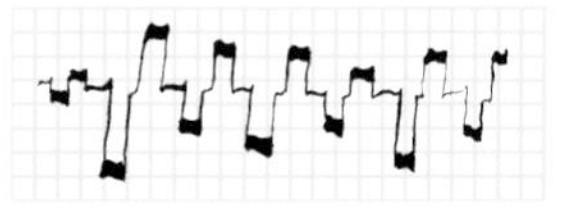

Diagram 3

The Segmental Electrogram allows us to see the suppressive effect of steroids at work. Normally after acupuncture stimulation the deflections on the recording widen, indicating the measure of stimulation that has been absorbed by the energy pathways. The recordings illustrated in diagrams 1 and 2 are taken from patients who are on steroid medication and who have just received acupuncture stimulation. Each graph shows a virtually straight line recording. Patients with severe allergies and who do not experience the dai chi needle sensation produce similar straight line recordings after acupuncture treatment. This is a very different picture from diagram 3, which shows the effect of acupuncture on someone who is neither on steroid treatment nor eating food to which he or she is allergic.

It is my firm view that many people who suffer from severe allergies end up with a suppressed immune system. Their reaction to energy stimulation therapies such as acupuncture is exactly the same as if they were receiving immuno-suppressive medication.

Since the objective of acupuncture treatment is to recharge and rebalance the energy-hormonal system, allergies can make it difficult for the therapy to have its desired affect.

Chapter Thirteen

Towards Good Health

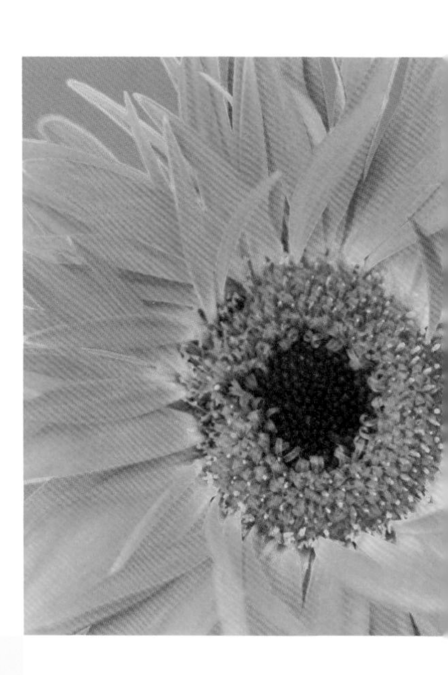

This book was written to help people back to good health using allergy testing and Five Element acupuncture. There is however, a right and a wrong time to use these systems.

I believe many of the thousands of people who visit GPs' surgeries every day would be better served by the treatments listed in this book. However, unavoidably, there will also be cases of acute and very serious illness – pneumonia, TB, cancer, and the like – for which the technology at the disposal of hospitals is essential for diagnosis and treatment. Such cases require immediate attention and the local GP and hospital are the appropriate places to seek help.

Anyone who develops an acute condition should first visit a GP or local hospital for an accurate diagnosis. This is particularly important where it is a baby or young child who is ill. Then, safe in the knowledge that the condition is not life-threatening, you have time to consider your options.

This book, however, has focused on the treatment of chronic, not acute, conditions. In these cases, once a diagnosis has been made and treatment options have been considered, a person may decide not to pursue the orthodox treatment approach immediately.

At the same time it is helpful and advisable for people who decide to follow an alternative course of treatment to keep in contact with their GP and hospital. The doctor who is genuinely interested and concerned about your health will be happy to hear of your progress and will generally be pleased to give assistance or advice, especially on matters relating to medication. A second opinion from someone who knows you and your medical history is always useful.

Eastern Versus Western Medicine

There is one fundamental difference of approach between Eastern and Western medicine. Western medicine considers that the majority of diseases are caused by external factors such as bacteria and viruses, and treatment involves the use of drugs such as antibiotics and steroids to exterminate these agents.

Eastern medicine recognises these external factors but believes that they cause a problem only when the person concerned has a weakened resistance. Emphasis is placed on finding out what has weakened a person's resistance, and then on applying a system of treatment focused on re-building and strengthening that resistance. Because of the holistic nature of Eastern medicine its treatments can take time to take effect. They are accordingly less appropriate in acute situations, which are potentially life-threatening.

Louis Pasteur

In his book *The Diseases of Civilisation* (36) Brian Inglis points out the incompleteness of the "germ theory" as proposed by Louis Pasteur. Observers of Pasteur's time noted that germs flourish best where the host is accommodating. On his deathbed, according to a friend who was with him, Pasteur himself admitted that he had made errors of judgment, and said, "The germ is nothing; the terrain is everything."

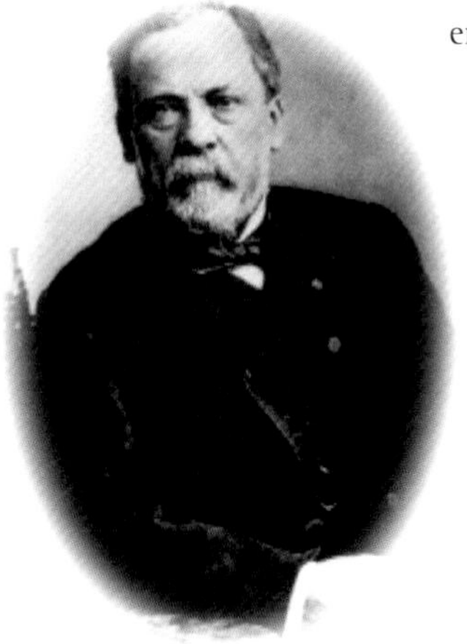

The theory upon which millions of prescriptions for antibiotics are written worldwide every year was thus an incomplete theory. By the time of Pasteur's death, however, the pharmaceutical industry had already grown huge, making vast fortunes from the sale of antibiotics and other drugs developed as a result of this germ theory of disease.

The Terrain is Everything

It is not that the germ theory is completely wrong. It is just that too much importance has been ascribed to it. If you develop pneumonia it will be likely to kill you if you do not take an antibiotic. However, preoccupation with the germ theory has resulted in the germ being regarded as the primary cause of all of our ills. This has led to the overuse of antibiotics, which in turn causes the weakening of people's immune systems and makes them increasingly vulnerable to further bacterial and viral attack. The result is ever more prescribing of antibiotics, and, before long, people caught in a downward spiral of infection and re-infection.

The preoccupation with germs and viruses has blinded Western medicine to the bigger, underlying picture concerned with immunity and the individual's constitution. When the viral epidemics of winter arrive, certain people are affected and others, living and working in the same environment, are not. If germs and viruses were the only triggers of these conditions, all people sharing an environment would be affected equally.

We come, then, to the central question: What is it that creates the terrain that incubates bacteria and viruses?

The answer to this begins with the stress and worry that result from all the difficult and trying life situations in which we find ourselves. Stress and worry result in poor digestion, which in turn leads to undigested foods fermenting and putrefying in the intestines. The resulting poisons get into the bloodstream and travel throughout the body, poisoning organs which are genetically vulnerable. A person from a long line of TB or bronchitis sufferers may have inherited a genetic weakness in the lungs and, if so, the toxins will congregate there. A person with a family history of arthritis will be likely to show a weakness in the joints, and the toxins will make these their point of attack. This poisoning of the body causes antibodies to be released, which trigger inflammatory reactions at the site concerned. In each case the person ends up with a toxic body, irritated by inflammatory antibody-induced reactions, and also emotionally depleted because of all the worry and stress. This is the terrain, the happy breeding ground, for bacteria and viruses.

Final Thoughts

If we are going to establish the very best health care system we can, ordinary people will have to start to question every aspect of the obvious inconsistencies in the current system. There is always an alternative and a second opinion. It is imperative that people become informed so that they can question the doctrines of the complementary and orthodox medical professions alike.

Sorting out your health is not impossible and it does not have to cost the earth. If you have an allergy-related condition, find out what your allergies are. Most people have relatively few primary allergies and the detection and avoidance of these is usually sufficient to bring about a dramatic recovery in health.

The additional treatment approach that I use to assist allergy sufferers is one which is directed towards assisting and supporting the nervous system. The Five Element acupuncture approach aims to release emotional blocks from within the nervous system. It also has the potential to strengthen the nervous system and thus enable it to resist future emotional stresses more efficiently. As a result of treatment, people feel emotionally stronger within themselves. They are uplifted and in a general way much better able to cope with life. As life's burdens are lifted from them, their immune system stops producing allergy reactions. The only reason it produced such reactions in the first place was to inform them of their body's distress.

Many of the treatment approaches promoted by the scientific community are designed principally to suppress the reactions of the immune system. The body is thus denied an opportunity for emotional release, and as a result, the person's distress remains locked within.

Dampening down these natural responses only ever gives short-term relief and is in general accompanied by undesirable side-effects.

The irony of it all is that many of you, who perhaps sat at your breakfast table this morning demoralised as a result of your present medical condition, bewildered as a result of the utter failure of science to ease your plight, and at a complete loss as to what you should do next, will be very surprised to find that the cause of all your distress has been on that plate in front of you, looking at you straight in the face, all this time.

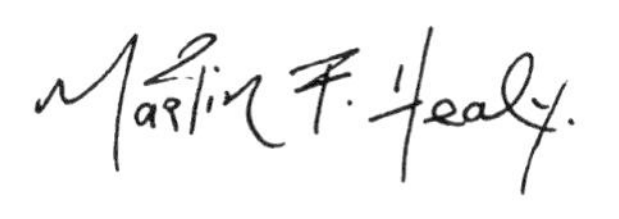

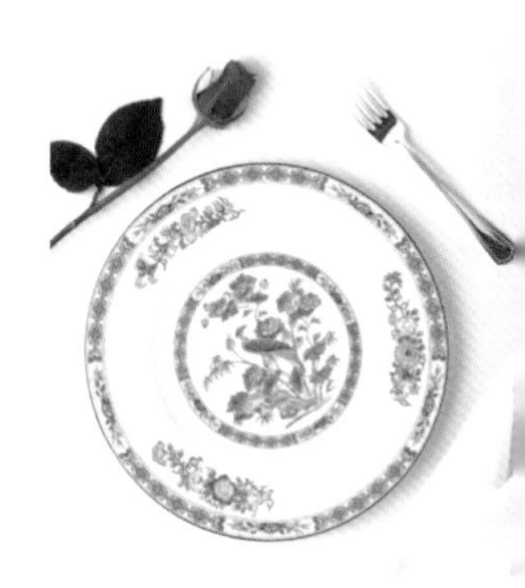

Appendix 1

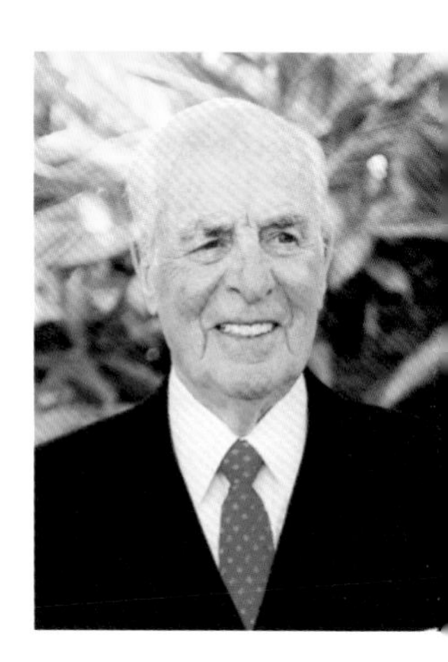

Professor J.R. Worsley

A style of acupuncture with a very strong and almost exclusively emotional focus, has become known as Five Element Acupuncture. One man who did more than any other to bring this particular style to the Western world is Professor J.R. Worsley. Worsley is an Englishman who studied acupuncture in the early 1960s in Taiwan and other parts of the Far East. After he returned from the East, Worsley spent many years putting together aspects of the complex web of human nature to formulate the Five Element approach. The system is directed towards touching the emotional aspect of the patient's life. He founded the College of Traditional Acupuncture, in England, to teach this style of treatment.

Worsley's emphasis runs in tandem with the work of other Western physicians of the last century who were developing treatment systems focused upon relieving their patients' stress and worry. Most influential in this field were the German homeopath and physician Dr. Samuel Hahnemann and the English herbalist and physician Dr. Edward Bach (*see* Appendix 2).

There are many different styles of acupuncture, each with a different emphasis. It is not that any one is superior to another, as different styles suit different conditions; but I believe that the Five Element style, as taught by Worsley, is particularly appropriate for people who have allergies.

Appendix 2

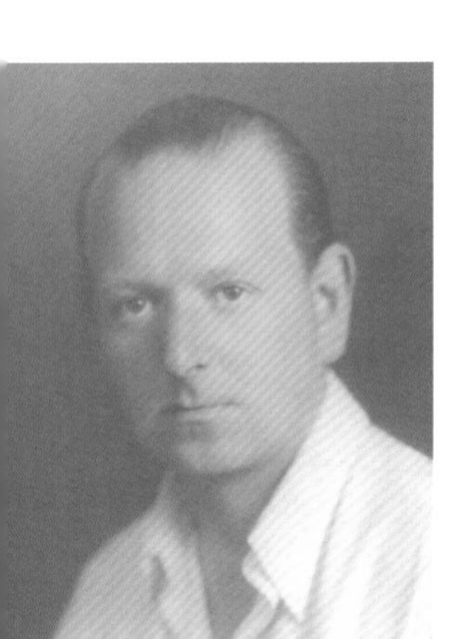

Dr. Edward Bach *(physician and herbalist) (1886–1936)*

At the turn of the last century Edward Bach, physician, pathologist, bacteriologist and herbalist, recognised that many diseases stemmed from bowel toxicity.

At University College Hospital, London, after many years working in general medicine, Bach studied bacteriology. There he discovered that certain intestinal germs, which up until then had been considered of little or no importance, were closely connected with many long-standing and chronic diseases.

He found that particular germs were present in the intestines of all his patients who suffered chronic disease. Further investigations showed that these same germs were also present in healthy individuals, but were far more prolific in people who were suffering with active disease. He began to investigate these bacteria, the relationship they bore to particular diseases, and why they were there in such great numbers.

Bach began to understand that the primary cause of this toxicity within the bowel was diet. He noticed that people who ate a healthy diet had very different faeces from those who ate an unhealthy diet. He discovered that there was a definite relationship between the disease condition and the numbers of toxic bacteria present in the bowel. In virtually all cases, as soon as the faecal bacteria start to decline the disease condition starts to disappear. The reverse is also true, in that as soon as the bacterial count starts to increase, the condition begins to worsen.

Bach found that these abnormal bowel bacteria were not in themselves disease-forming. Their danger lies in the toxins that they slowly produce. It is this prolonged, continued action which gradually and insidiously lowers the vitality of the individual, and this increases the person's susceptibility to both acute and chronic disease.

Bach wrote in his notes of this period that the human subject becomes infected very early in life, and so commonly are these organisms found in adults and children that many laboratories regard their presence as reasonably normal. However, the dramatic improvement in health that is associated with their removal proves that they are far from normal inhabitants.

After many years of investigating the phenomenon of bowel bacteria, Bach failed to convince his medical colleagues of their relevance to medicine. He ultimately became disillusioned with Western medicine and abandoned it completely. He left the hospitals of London, and his Harley Street practice, and settled in Oxfordshire, where he dedicated his remaining years to the study of the true nature of disease. It was during those last years of his life in the countryside of Oxford that he came to understand clearly how worry and stress can exacerbate any medical condition. It was also during this period that he established the Edward Bach Centre (see illustration below) and developed the famous Bach Flower Remedies.

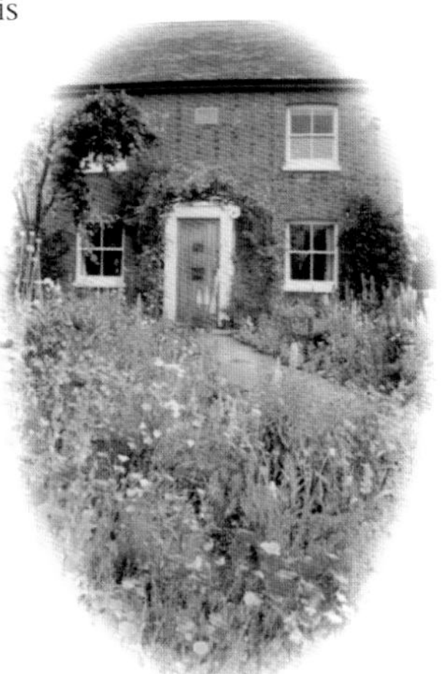

The Dr. Edward Bach Centre, Mount Vernon, Sotwell, Oxfordshire, England

Appendix 3

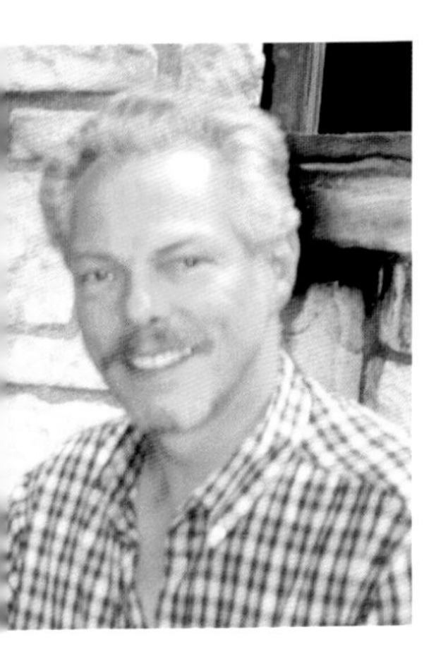

Simon Charles *(homoeopath and psychotherapist)*

Simon Charles is an Englishman who studied natural medicines in the 1970s. We worked together in London for a period where I observed his particular expertise in dealing with patients with chronic stress.

In general, the stress we experience can be regarded as being of an acute or chronic nature. Acute stresses are usually short-lived episodes, are triggered by life events such as bereavement, relationship break-up and all the other heartaches and disappointments which are part and parcel of normal living, along with the everyday stresses of work overload, deadlines, traffic etc. People who suffer with allergies appear to be more sensitive to the effects of these stresses. In such cases, acupuncture appears to be the fastest and most supportive way of getting the person back onto an even keel.

Chronic stress is different, being generally associated with deep-rooted negative beliefs and fears. Working with a skilled and experienced psychotherapist or counsellor is often the best way of dealing with such problems.

References

(1) Awazuhara H., Kawai H., et al. (1997) Major allergens in soybean and clinical significance of IgG4 antibodies investigated by IgE- and IgG4-immunoblotting with sera from soybean-sensitive patients, *Clin Exp Allergy*, 27, 3, pp.325–32

Beauvais F., Hieblot C., et al. (1990) Bimodal IgG4-mediated human basophil activation: Role of eosinophils, *J Immunol*, 144, 10, pp.3881–90

Berrens L. and Homedes I.B. (1991) Relationship between IgE and IgG antibodies in type I allergy, *Allerg Immunol*, 37, 3–4, pp.131–7

Cavataio F., Iacono G., et al. (1996) Gastroesophageal reflux associated with cow's milk allergy in infants: Which diagnostic examinations are useful?, *Am J Gastroenterol*, 91, 6, pp.1215–20

Cohen G.A., Hartman G., et al. (1985) Severe anaemia and chronic bronchitis associated with a markedly elevated specific IgG to cow's milk protein, *Ann Allergy*, 55, 1, pp.38–40

Firer M.A., Hosking C.S., et al. (1981) Effect of antigen load on development of milk antibodies in infants allergic to milk, *Br Med J*, 283, 6293, pp.693–6

Halpern G.M. and Scott J.R. (1987) Non-IgE antibody mediated mechanisms in food allergy, *Ann Allergy*, 58, 1, pp.14–27

Hofman T. (1995) IgE and IgG antibodies in children with food allergy, *Rocz Akad Med Bialymst*, 40, 3, pp.468–73

Iikura Y., Akimoto, K., et al. (1989) How to prevent allergic disease: I. Study of specific IgE, IgG, and IgG 4 antibodies in serum of pregnant mothers, cord blood, and infants, *Int Arch Allergy Appl Immunol*, 88, 1–2, pp.250–2

Marinkovich V. (1996) Specific IgG antibodies as markers of adverse reactions to foods, *Monogr Allergy*, 32, pp.221–5

McDonald P.J., Goldblum R.M., et al. (1984) Food protein-induced enterocolitis: Altered antibody response to ingested antigen, *Pediatr Res*, 18, 8, pp.751–5

Nakagawa T. (1991) The role of IgG subclass antibodies in the clinical response to immunotherapy in allergic disease, *Clin Exp Allergy*, 21, 3, pp.289–96

Nakagawa T., Mukoyama T., et al. (1986) Egg white-specific IgE and IgG4 antibodies in atopic children, *Ann Allergy*, 57, 5, pp.359–62

Parish W.E. (1970) Short-term anaphylactic IgG antibodies in human sera, *Lancet*, 2, 7673, pp.591–2

Shakib F., Brown H.M., et al. (1986) Study of IgG sub-class antibodies in patients with milk intolerance, *Clin Allergy*, 16, 5, pp.451–8

Taylor C.J., Hendrickse R.G., et al. (1988) Detection of cow's milk protein intolerance by an enzyme-linked immunosorbent assay, *Acta Paediatr Scand*, 77, 1, pp.49–54

Trevino R.J. (1981) Immunologic mechanisms in the production of food sensitivities, *Laryngoscope*, 91, 11, pp.1913–36

(2) Roitt I.M., Brostoff J., et al. (1996) *Immunology*, 4th edn., London: Mosby

(3) Brighton W.D. (1980) Frequency of occurrences of IgG (S–TS), *Clin Allergy*, 10, 1, pp.97–100

(4) Brostoff J. and Gamlin L. (1992) *A Complete Guide to Food Allergy and Intolerance*, London: Bloomsbury

(5) Walzer M. (1941) Allergy of the abdominal organs, *J Lab Clin Med*, 26, pp.1867–77
Brummer M. and Walzer M. (1928) Absorption of undigested proteins in human beings: The absorption of unaltered fish protein in adults, *Arch Intern Med*, 42, pp.173–9

Host A. (1994) Cow's milk protein allergy and intolerance in infancy, *Pediatr Allergy Immunol*, 5, pp.5–36